Publisher: Henry Plociennik
Edited by: Christine Richter
Design: Susan Kinealy

Acknowledgements: For kindly giving permission to use recipes and photographs from the UK Edition of The Make It Simple Cookbook by Ann Page-Wood, published by New English Library, we acknowledge the use of the following photographed recipes on pages:11,15,19,23,27,43,51,63,67,71,79,83,87.91,95,103,107,111, 115,119,123.
Additional food photography: Quentin Bacon.
Food stylist for additional photography: Vo Bacon.

National Library of Australia Card number and ISBN 1 86292 006 0.

Published by Compass Publishing Co Pty Limited, 155 Castlereagh Street, Sydney, NSW, 2000. Australia.
Published by arrangement with NAL PENGUIN INC. New York, New York.

Typeset by Photoset Computer Service Pty Limited, Sydney, NSW, Australia.

Printed by: Kyodo Printing, Singapore.

Cover Picture: *Fruit rings, (page 110).*

WEIGHT WATCHERS®

KEEP IT SIMPLE

—————— STEP-BY-STEP ——————

C O O K B O O K

COMPASS PUBLISHING CO PTY LIMITED
155 Castlereagh Street,
Sydney, NSW,2000. Australia.

Published by arrangement with
NAL PENGUIN INC. New York, New York.

PUBLISHER'S NOTE

Welcome to one of the most exciting new cookbooks in the Weight Watchers publishing program.

Our *Keep It Simple, Step-By-Step Cookbook* is, as the name implies, a recipe book which has been developed to meet the needs of the busy lifestyle of today.

The recipes also reflect our changing tastes and eating habits. They have been designed to give quick, positive results for those on the Weight Watchers program.

It is a fact of life that we are basically creatures of habit and tend to cook and eat the same types of foods.

The Weight Watchers weight-loss program has been developed to provide as much flexibility and variety in food and recipes as is possible to help overcome boredom.

To support and reinforce that program we have developed this *Keep It Simple Cookbook* which features easy to prepare meals which are uncomplicated, and more importantly, which are refreshingly satisfying to people on diets.

They have been developed to simplify demands on you in the kitchen but still enable you to create dinners which the entire family will enjoy.

Our recipes reinforce the message that staying on the Weight Watchers program and losing weight need not be dull.

CONTENTS

INTRODUCTION

Weight Watchers promotes a weight-loss program that is more than a diet — rather it is a proven program to help revise eating habits, particularly bad habits.

Weight Watchers is the largest organisation of its kind in the world. Its expertise and success in the weight-loss field is recognised by leading nutritionists and the medical profession. With its four-way approach to weight control — the Food Plan, Self-Management Plan, Exercise Plan and Group Support System — Weight Watchers also offers versatility and flexibility.

The program's versatility and flexibility allows for a wide range of culinary delights and hence cookbooks such as this one can offer a wide range of recipes from savory appetisers to delicious main meals and tasty sweet treats.

ABOUT OUR RECIPES

The recipes in the *Keep It Simple Cookbook* were developed mainly as one or two serving dishes, which will be of special interest to Weight Watchers members. The serving suggestions for recipes cooked from this book will mean that it will be easier for members to keep to the program.

When developing the recipes, we ensured that the high standard of healthy nutritional values expected in the balanced Weight Watchers food plan would be maintained.

Each recipe comes with Weight Watchers exchange information which tells you how one serving from that dish fits into the program. If you make any changes in the recipes, please be sure to adjust the exchange information accordingly.

Each recipe also gives the exchanges for Protein, Bread, Vegetables, Fat, Fruit, Milk and Optional Kilojoules.

Photographed recipes may vary as to the number of servings shown. Please see recipes for exact serving information.

METHOD

The method in which the recipes have been developed will be of special interest to Weight Watchers members. In any recipe of more than one serving, it is important to mix the ingredients well and divide the mixture evenly so that every portion has an equal amount of each ingredient.

Where liquid and solid parts have to be divided evenly, drain the liquid, set aside and follow procedure above for remaining ingredients; add equal amounts of the liquid to each portion.

When selecting fruits or juices other than fresh, choose those with no sugar added. Use only low-fat yoghurt in natural or reduced-kilojoule flavors.

Reduced-kilojoule jams contain 10 kJ per teaspoon, unless otherwise indicated.

WEIGHING

The recipes in this book were developed using Australian Standard Measures. The lists of ingredients have also been simplified, especially when giving quantities.

It is important to weigh and measure ingredients accurately to achieve the best results. This also ensures that you have the correct quantities for your exchanges.

Always use accurate spoon and cup measures.

While many parts of the Weight Watchers program call for teaspoon measures, often the number of teaspoons required in a recipe is high. In order to avoid mistakes being made when measuring out multiple quantities of teaspoons, we have changed the quantity to tablespoons and/or cup measures when the teaspoon count exceeds three. Similarly cup measures are given when the required number of tablespoons exceeds three.

(For Australian readers, one teaspoon equals 5mL and one tablespoon is equal to four teaspoons, 20mL. In New Zealand, one tablespoon is equal to three teaspoons, 15mL.)

To measure liquids, use a standard glass or clear plastic measuring cup. Always read the markings at eye level and make sure the container is placed on a level surface before you take the reading. To measure less than ¼ cup, use standard measuring spoons.

To measure dry ingredients, use metal or plastic measuring cups that come in sets of four: ¼ cup; ⅓ cup; ½ cup; and 1 cup. Spoon the ingredients into the cup, then level with the straight edge of a knife or metal spatula. To measure less than ¼ cup, use standard measuring spoons and, unless directed otherwise, level as for measuring cup.

FATS AND OILS

When vegetable oil is called for, oils such as safflower, sunflower, soybean, corn, cottonseed, peanut, or any of these combined may be used. In some recipes, Chinese sesame oil and olive oil, because of their distinctive flavors, have been specifically indicated.

To reduce the amount of fat used in cooking and therefore reduce the kilojoule intake, it is worth lining baking sheets and pans with non-stick papers instead of greasing them. Also consider using non-stick fry pans.

FRUIT

Unless specified, fresh fruit has been used in recipes, but frozen or canned fruit packed in natural juice, with no sugar added, may be substituted when appropriate. However, it may be necessary to adjust cooking times accordingly.

VEGETABLES

We have used fresh vegetables unless otherwise indicated. If you substitute frozen or canned vegetables, it may be necessary to adjust cooking times accordingly.

MEAT AND POULTRY

Always buy the leanest possible meat. It is often best to buy meat, remove any visible fat and mince it yourself to avoid fatty mince. Meat and poultry skin should be removed, whenever possible, before cooking.

Cook all meat except offal and poultry, on a rack under the grill. Always bake or roast meat on a rack and never use the fat that runs out in gravies or sauces. All the weights of meat given in the lists of ingredients are for the uncooked meat trimmed of all fat.

SEASONINGS

The herbs used it these recipes are dried unless otherwise indicated. If you are substituting fresh herbs, use approximately four times the amount of dried (e.g., 1 teaspoon chopped fresh basil instead of ¼ teaspoon dried basil leaves). If you are substituting ground (powdered) herbs for dried leaves, use approximately half the amount of dried (e.g., ¼ teaspoon ground thyme instead of ½ teaspoon dried thyme leaves).

Spices. If you are substituting fresh spices for ground, generally use approximately eight times the amount of ground (e.g., 1 teaspoon crushed ginger root instead of ⅛ teaspoon of ground ginger).

Generally, dried herbs and spices should not be kept for more than a year. Date the container at the time of purchase and check occasionally for potency. Usually, if the herb or spice is aromatic, it is still potent; if the aroma has diminished, the recipe may require a larger amount of the seasoning.

EGGS AND CHEESE

Eggs are probably the most versatile ingredient in the kitchen. They supply essential proteins, vitamins and minerals and can be cooked and served on their own or used to enrich a variety of dishes. Basically a solidified form of milk, cheese is rich in protein and minerals but, according to the type of cheese, may provide a considerable amount of fat. There are hundreds of different cheeses but in this book they are divided into two basic categories — hard and low-fat.

SPANISH OMELETTE

SERVES 1

This is a meal in itself. Use a non-stick or heavy-based omelette pan, as the omelette is turned to cook the underside and not folded over. You may find it easier to slide the omelette onto a plate, then invert it back into the pan.

1 teaspoon vegetable or olive oil
¼ medium green capsicum, seeded and chopped
¼ medium red capsicum, seeded and chopped
4 shallots or ½ small onion, chopped
1 medium tomato, peeled and chopped
75g peeled cooked potato, cubed
¼ cup cooked peas
2 eggs, beaten
1½ tablespoons water
pinch mixed herbs
pinch each salt and pepper

1. Heat the oil in a small omelette pan. Add the green and red capsicum and shallots or onion and stir-fry for about 4 minutes or until soft. Add the tomato, potato and peas.

2. In a bowl whisk together all the remaining ingredients.

3. Pour the egg mixture over the vegetables, stir and cook over a moderate heat, shaking the pan occasionally and easing the edge of the omelette away from the pan.

4. When the underside is golden brown, slide onto a plate using a fish slice. Turn upside down back into the pan and continue cooking until the other side is golden brown.

5. Slide the thick omelette onto a warm serving plate.

EXCHANGES PER SERVING:
Protein 2
Bread 1
Vegetable 3½
Fat 1

Spanish Omelette, pictured at end of Step 3 in method.

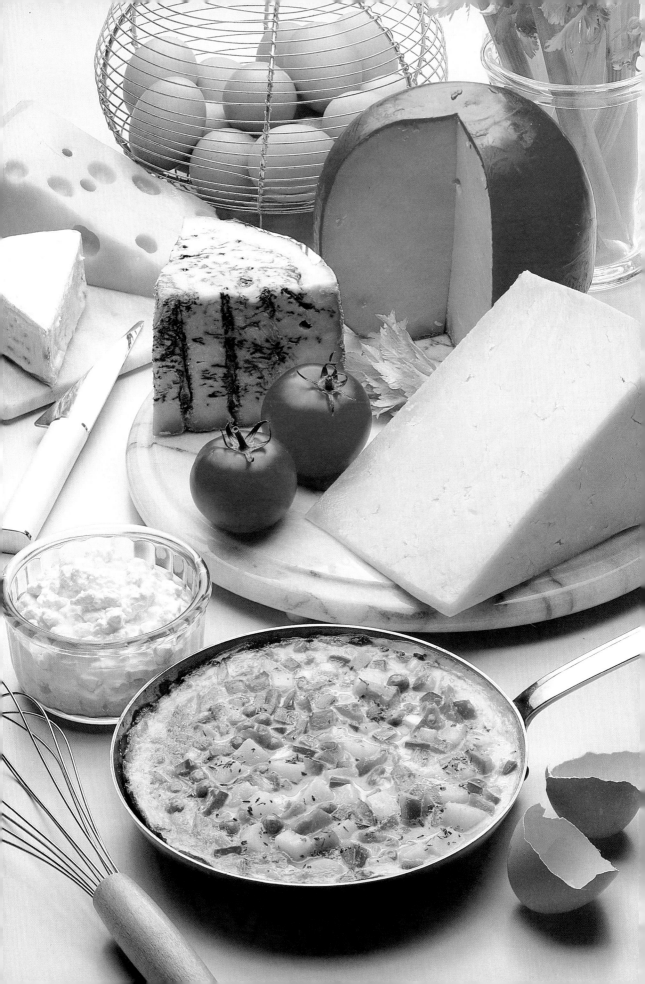

PEPPER FRITTATA

SERVES 1

A frittata is cooked very slowly over a low heat, the opposite method to cooking an omelette, and when the base is golden brown the pan is transferred to a grill to complete the cooking. It is served whole, not folded over. A crisp salad makes an ideal accompaniment.

1½ teaspoons vegetable or olive oil
¼ medium green capsicum, seeded and chopped
¼ medium red capsicum, seeded and chopped
1 tablespoon chopped shallots
1 small clove garlic, finely chopped
2 eggs
1½ tablespoons water
30g tasty cheese, finely grated
pinch each salt and pepper

1. Heat ½ teaspoon of oil in a small omelette pan. Add the green and red capsicum, shallots and garlic and stir-fry 4-5 minutes until soft.

2. Beat the eggs and water together in a bowl, add the stir-fried vegetables, about half the cheese and the salt and pepper.

3. Add the remaining oil to the omelette pan, cook over a low heat, swirl around the pan.

4. Pour the egg mixture into the pan, turn the heat down to low and cook very slowly without stirring for 10-12 minutes until the underside is golden. Remove from the heat, sprinkle with the remaining cheese.

5. Transfer to a preheated grill and cook until the cheese has melted and is bubbling. Slide onto a warm serving plate.

EXCHANGES PER SERVING:
Protein 3
Vegetable 1⅛
Fat 1½

BAKED MACARONI CHEESE

SERVES 2

Try this simple but delicious way of making macaroni cheese.

2 teaspoons polyunsaturated margarine
$\frac{1}{2}$ cup chopped onion
$1\frac{1}{2}$ cups cooked elbow macaroni
120g Cheddar cheese, grated
30g sliced leg ham, chopped
$\frac{3}{4}$ cup evaporated skim milk
1 egg
$\frac{1}{4}$ teaspoon salt
$\frac{1}{8}$ teaspoon pepper
$\frac{1}{4}$ teaspoon paprika

1. Heat margarine in a small pan, add onion and stir-fry until translucent but not brown.

2. Spread half of the macaroni over base of medium casserole dish. Top with half of the cheese, ham and sautéed onion. Repeat layers.

3. Preheat oven to 180°C. Combine milk, egg, salt and pepper in a mixing bowl, pour over macaroni mixture and sprinkle with paprika.

4. Bake for about 20 minutes, until hot and bubbly.

EXCHANGES PER SERVING:
Protein 3
Bread $1\frac{1}{2}$
Vegetable $\frac{1}{2}$
Fat 1
Milk $\frac{3}{4}$

CHEESE SOUFFLÉ

SERVES 2

This is a basic soufflé recipe. The cheese may be omitted and replaced with 90g finely chopped ham or a mixture of 45g cheese and 45g ham. Don't be tempted to add too much filling or the soufflé will be heavy. Always serve soufflés immediately.

1 tablespoon polyunsaturated margarine
1 tablespoon plain flour
½ cup skim milk
3 eggs, separated
45g Cheddar cheese, grated
45g Parmesan cheese, grated
1 tablespoon chopped chives or shallots
½ teaspoon salt
pinch each pepper and powered mustard

1. Use 1 teaspoon of the margarine to grease a 15cm soufflé dish.

2. Heat the remaining margarine in a medium saucepan, add the flour and cook over a low heat for 1-2 minutes, stirring all the time.

3. Remove from the heat and gradually blend in the milk. Bring to the boil, stirring continuously, boil for 1 minute.

4. Allow to cool a little then beat in the egg yolks, cheeses, chives or shallots, ¼ teaspoon of the salt, pepper and mustard.

5. Preheat oven to 180°C. Whisk the egg whites with remaining salt until soft peaks form. Lightly fold them into the cheese sauce using a tablespoon. Transfer the mixture to the soufflé dish and bake for about 35 minutes until golden brown, well risen and just set. Serve immediately.

EXCHANGES PER SERVING:
Protein 3
Fat 2
Milk ¼
100 Kilojoules Optional Exchange

Cheese Soufflé.

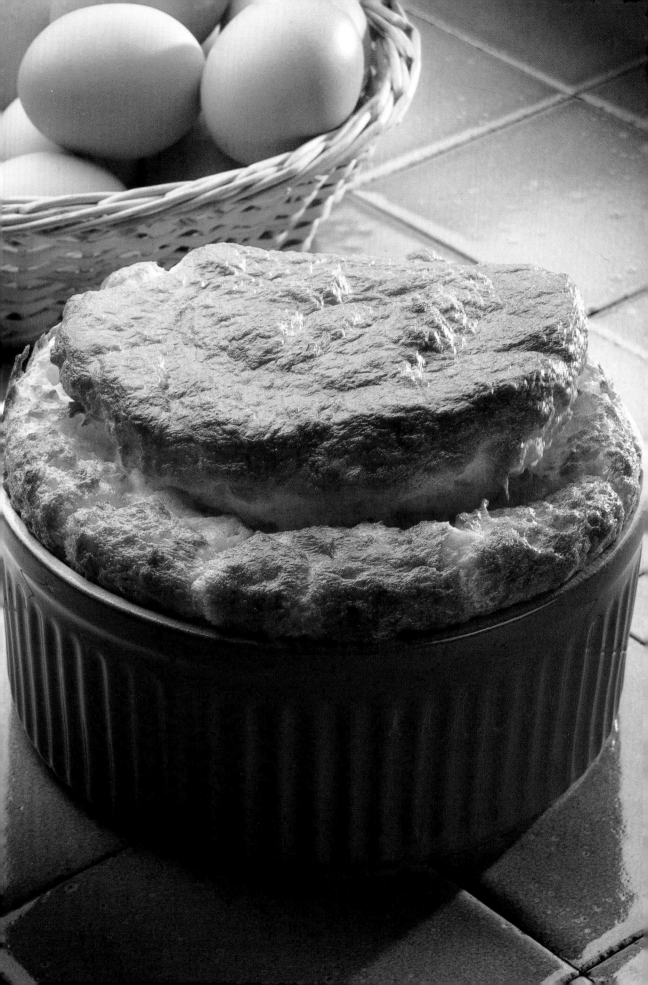

CHEESY MEXICAN CHIPS

A great cheesy snack with a Mexican flavor, pictured on page 31.

½ teaspoon polyunsaturated margarine
25g corn chips (P.C.Series:Parties)
30g grated Cheddar cheese
2 teaspoons chilli sauce
½ teaspoon paprika

1. Preheat oven to 180°C. Grease the base of a 20cm spring-form pan with the margarine. Pile corn chips in centre of prepared pan. Sprinkle cheese over corn chips.

2. Bake for 3-5 minutes or until cheese has melted. Remove from oven and top with chilli sauce and sprinkle with paprika. Serve immediately.

EXCHANGES PER SERVING:
Protein ½
305 Kilojoules Optional Exchange

STUFFED EGGS

SERVES 2

This is a simple, basic recipe which you can adapt to suit your own tastes. Try adding 30g minced ham or drained, canned flaked tuna to the stuffing mixture, and serve on a bed of shredded lettuce. These variations will increase Protein Exchanges to 3.

4 hard-cooked eggs, shelled
60g cottage or ricotta cheese
3 teaspoons mayonnaise
2 teaspoons chopped chives
½ teaspoon mashed anchovy
pinch salt
pinch paprika
sprigs of parsley to garnish
2 lettuce leaves

1. Halve the eggs lengthwise and scoop out the yolks into a bowl.

2. Mash the egg yolks with the cottage or ricotta cheese, mayonnaise, chives, anchovy and salt.

3. Either pile the stuffing back into the egg whites or place in a piping bag fitted with a 1.25cm star nozzle and pipe into the whites.

4. Dust each egg with paprika and garnish with sprigs of parsley. Serve on lettuce leaves.

EXCHANGES PER SERVING:
Protein 2½
Vegetable ¼
Fat 1½
15 Kilojoules Optional Exchange

CHEESE AND YOGHURT MOUSSE

Almost any soft fruit can be used as a topping for this mousse, not only the kiwi fruit and strawberries featured here.

120g cottage cheese
1½ tablespoons castor sugar
few drops of vanilla essence
1½ teaspoons gelatine
1½ tablespoons hot water
½ cup low-fat natural yoghurt
2 egg whites
pinch salt
1 cup strawberries
1 large kiwi fruit, sliced

1. Beat the cottage cheese, sugar and vanilla essence together.

2. In a bowl sprinkle the gelatine over the hot water, stir. Stand the container in a saucepan of simmering water until the gelatine has dissolved.

3. Gradually beat the yoghurt into the cottage cheese mixture.

4. Stir a little of the cottage cheese and yoghurt into the dissolved gelatine, pour into the cottage cheese mixture and mix well.

5. Whisk the egg whites with the salt until soft peaks form. Fold into the cheese mixture using a metal spoon.

6. Divide between two wide dessert dishes, cover and refrigerate until set.

7. Set aside 2 whole strawberries; cut remaining berries in half lengthwise. Decorate each mousse with half each of the kiwi fruit and strawberry halves. Garnish centre of each with whole berry.

EXCHANGES PER SERVING:
Protein 1
Fruit 1
Milk ½
400 Kilojoules Optional Exchange

Cheese and Yoghurt Mousse.

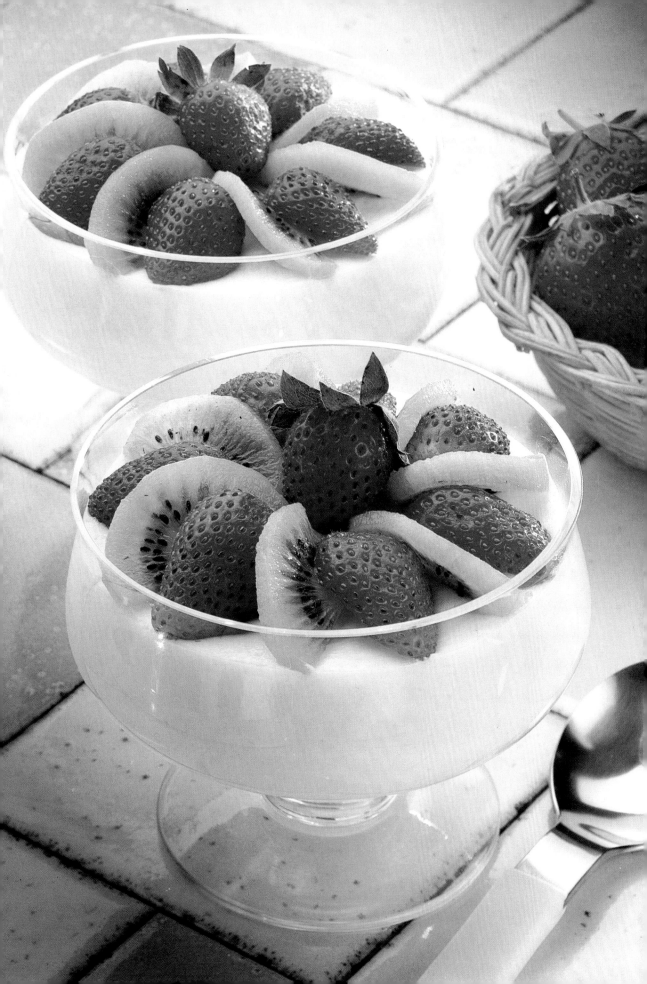

CREPES

Crepes take a lot of practice to make well. They should be very thin, not thick and stodgy. Use as the basis for a dessert such as Brandied Apricots Flambé (page 94) or stuffed with a savory filling such as Savory Mince (page 32).

½ cup plain flour
pinch salt
1 egg, beaten
¾ cup skim milk
2 teaspoons polyunsaturated margarine or vegetable oil

1. Sieve the flour and salt into a bowl, make a well in the centre, add the egg, and gradually beat or whisk in the milk. Put to one side.

2. Season an 18cm crepe pan. This will help to prevent the crepes sticking and reduce the amount of oil required for cooking them. Generously sprinkle salt over the base of the crepe pan, heat gently, tip out the salt, then wipe thoroughly with a pad of kitchen paper. Heat ½ teaspoon of margarine or oil in the pan and once again wipe around the pan.

3. Heat ⅛ of the remaining margarine or oil in the pan, pour in the batter while turning the pan so it thinly coats the base. Cook over moderate heat until the underside is golden, toss or turn over and cook the other side.

4. Transfer the cooked crepe to a plate, cover and keep warm in a low oven while repeating the procedure. This quantity should make 8 crepes.

EXCHANGES PER SERVING:
Protein ½
Bread 1½
Fat ½
Milk ¼
160 Kilojoules Optional Exchange

SWEET CHEESE PANCAKES

— SERVES 2 —

These little pancakes are served with honey or maple syrup, but if you prefer they could be sprinkled with the same quantity of castor sugar. This would provide the same Exchanges quoted below.

60g cottage or ricotta cheese
1 egg, separated
3 teaspoons plain flour
2 teaspoons castor sugar
2 teaspoons lemon juice
½ teaspoon finely grated lemon zest
pinch cinnamon
pinch salt
2 teaspoons vegetable oil
2 teaspoons honey or maple syrup

1. Cream the cottage or ricotta cheese and egg yolk in a bowl.

2. Mix in the flour, sugar, lemon juice, lemon zest and cinnamon.

3. In a separate bowl, whisk the egg white and salt until soft peaks form. Fold a little into the cheese mixture, using a metal spoon — this will lighten the mixture — then fold in the remaining egg white.

4. Heat 1 teaspoon of oil in a small pan, drop 2 tablespoons of the mixture into the hot oil and cook over a moderate heat until the underside is golden brown. Turn over and cook the other side.

5. Transfer the cooked pancakes to a warm plate. Heat the remaining oil and repeat the process with the rest of the mixture.

6. Serve the pancakes with the honey or maple syrup trickled over the top.

Exchanges per Serving:
Protein 1
Fat 1
275 Kilojoules Optional Exchange

MERINGUE BASKETS

SERVES 3

These meringue baskets can be filled with a variety of fresh fruits. Blueberries, pictured right, look particularly attractive.

1 egg white
pinch salt
¼ cup castor sugar
¾ cup blueberries

1. Line a baking sheet with baking paper.

2. Whisk the egg white and salt in a bowl until soft peaks form, add a tablespoon of castor sugar and continue whisking until the egg white forms peaks again.

3. Sprinkle in another tablespoon of castor sugar and whisk again until the same consistency is obtained. Fold in the remaining sugar with a metal spoon.

4. Preheat oven to 130°C. Transfer the meringue mixture to a piping bag fitted with a 1.25cm fluted nozzle. Pipe a circle about 7.5cm in diameter, pipe one or two rings on top of each other around the edge of the base circle to form a basket. There will be sufficient meringue to make three baskets.

5. Bake for about 3 hours until the meringues are firm and crisp but still white. If they begin to color open the oven door a little.

6. Cool baskets on a wire rack and either store in an airtight container or fill each with ¼ cup fruit and serve.

EXCHANGES PER SERVING:
Fruit ½
450 Kilojoules Optional Exchange

Meringue Baskets.

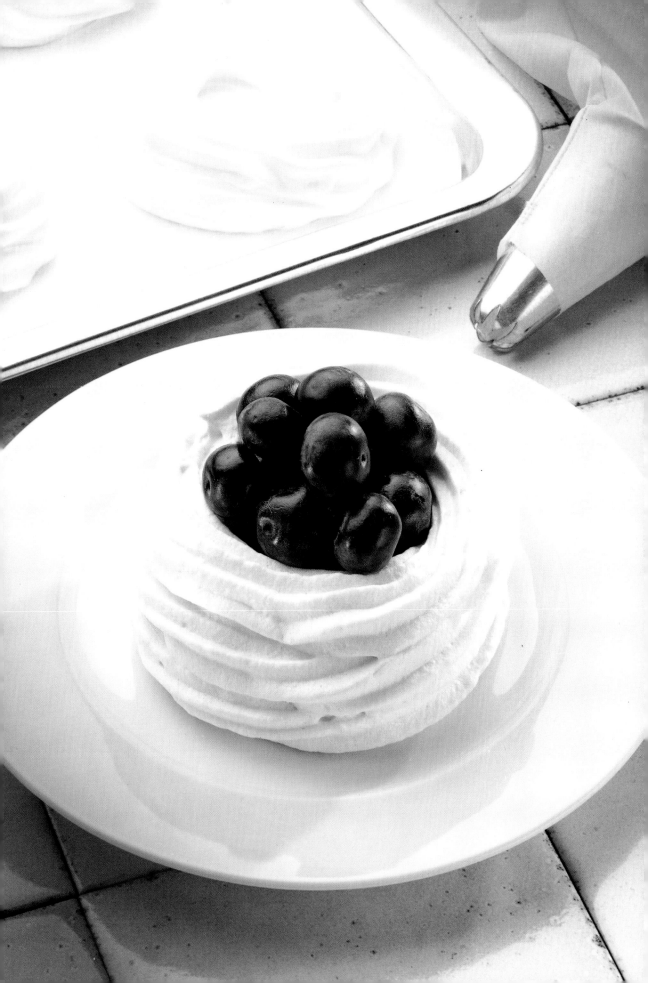

SULTANA CHEESE PUDDING

SERVES 2

Don't be surprised when the puddings rise during baking and then, as they cool, sink down and away from the sides of the ramekin. The pudding isn't meant to have the lightness of a soufflé. It is a delicious version of a cheesecake without the added kilojoules of a pastry or biscuit base.

½ teaspoon polyunsaturated margarine
120g ricotta cheese
1 egg, separated
20g sultanas
3 teaspoons castor sugar
grated zest of ½ a lemon
2 teaspoons lemon juice
pinch salt
To serve
1½ tablespoons whipped cream
2 slices of lemon

1. Grease two 150mL ramekins with the margarine.

2. Beat together the ricotta cheese, egg yolk, sultanas, sugar, lemon zest and lemon juice.

3. In a separate bowl, whisk the egg white and salt until soft peaks form.

4. Using a metal spoon, fold a tablespoon of egg white into the mixture, then fold in the remaining egg white.

5. Preheat oven to 160°C. Spoon the mixture into the prepared ramekins and bake for 25-30 minutes until set and beginning to brown. Leave to cool in the ramekins, then turn out onto the serving plates and leave until completely cold.

6. Just before serving, top each cheese pudding with a half of the cream and a twist of lemon.

EXCHANGES PER SERVING:
Protein 1½
Fruit ½
325 Kilojoules Optional Exchange

MEAT AND POULTRY

This is an excellent source of protein and therefore an important food to include in one's diet. Choose meat carefully — look for an even color and never buy meat which smells unpleasant. All weights for meat given in recipes are for meat purchased raw and trimmed of all fat. Meat must be grilled, baked or roasted on a rack, or boiled and then cooked.

STUFFED SAUSAGES AND CHILLI BEANS

SERVES 2

Spicy Mexican-style beans add flavor to the humble sausage.

2 x 120g beef sausages
120g drained, canned red kidney beans
1½ tablespoons tomato purée
⅛ teaspoon chilli powder
30g cream cheese
1½ teaspoons chopped fresh chives

1. Grill sausages on rack in grilling pan for 10-15 minutes or until done to taste.

2. While sausages are cooking, combine kidney beans, tomato purée and chilli powder in saucepan, stirring often until heated through.

3. Mix remaining ingredients in a bowl. Make a 1cm deep lengthwise slit in each sausage, fill each with half of the cream cheese mixture. Return to griller until cheese is lightly browned. Serve each sausage with half of the chilli bean mixture.

EXCHANGES PER SERVING:
Protein 4
Vegetable ⅛
200 Kilojoules Optional Exchange

Cheesy Mexican Chips (page 20);
Stuffed Sausages and Chilli Beans,
three servings pictured.

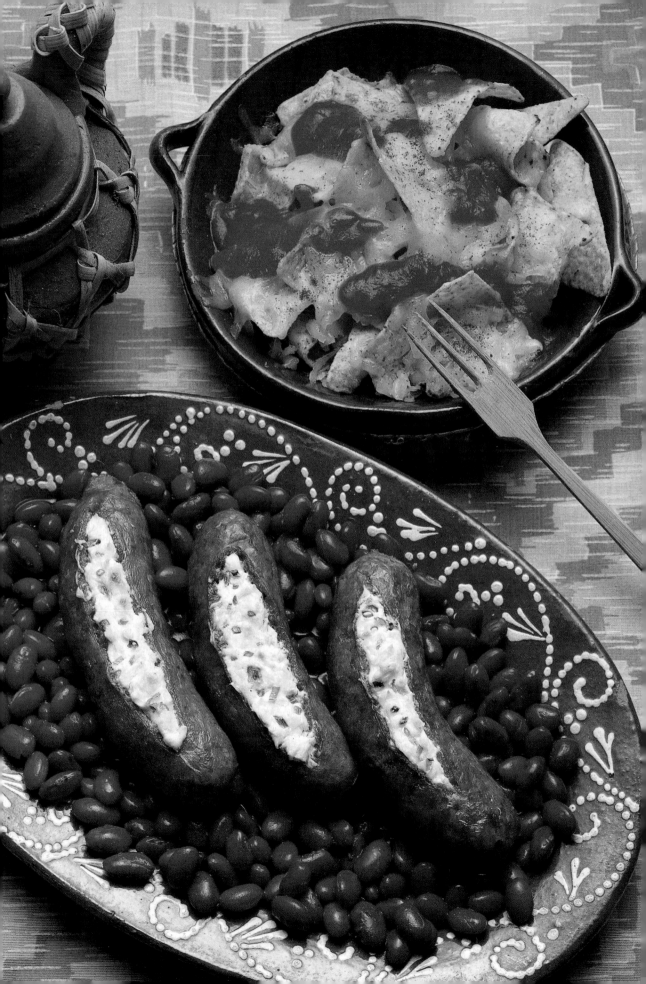

SAVORY MINCE

SERVES 2

This is a very simple, basic recipe. Add a chopped garlic clove and a bouquet garni for extra flavor. This mince makes a very nice filling for crepes (page 24).

230g minced veal
½ medium onion, chopped
½ medium carrot, diced
½ cup shelled peas
1 medium stick celery, sliced
½ cup mushrooms, sliced
3 teaspoons plain flour
1 beef stock cube, dissolved in ¾ cup water
¼ teaspoon mixed dried herbs
pinch each salt and pepper

1. Crumble the minced veal into a saucepan. Mix in the prepared vegetables.

2. Sprinkle in the flour and stir well. Gradually add the stock. Stir in herbs, salt and pepper.

3. Bring to the boil, stirring all the time. Cover, reduce the heat and simmer for 20 minutes, stirring occasionally.

EXCHANGES PER SERVING:
Protein 3
Vegetable 1¾
185 Kilojoules Optional Exchange

BEEF STROGANOFF

SERVES 2

Take care not to overcook the beef. After its initial grilling to remove the fat, it needs only a little extra cooking time.

2 teaspoons vegetable oil
1 medium onion, thinly sliced
1 cup button mushrooms, sliced
190g rump steak, grill until medium rare, slice thinly
¼ cup sour cream
pinch pepper

1. Heat the oil. Add the onion and sauté for 2-3 minutes until soft.

2. Add the mushrooms and steak and continue stirring over a moderate heat for about 4 minutes until the mushrooms and steak are cooked through.

3. Remove from the heat, stir in the sour cream and pepper and serve.

EXCHANGES PER SERVING:
Protein 2½
Vegetable 2
Fat 1
280 Kilojoules Optional Exchange

SAN CHOY BOW

—————————— SERVES 2 ——————————

Enjoy this favorite Chinese dish and still stay on the program.

150g minced veal
20g drained, canned water chestnuts, sliced
2 small Chinese mushrooms, soaked, drained and chopped
2 teaspoons chopped shallots
½ teaspoon soy sauce
¼ teaspoon each grated fresh ginger and crushed garlic
¼ teaspoon each sesame oil, dry sherry and oyster sauce
½ teaspoon vegetable oil
2 medium lettuce leaves
2 shallots for garnish

1. Combine all ingredients except vegetable oil, lettuce and garnish in a bowl. Cover and refrigerate for at least 1 hour.

2. Heat vegetable oil in medium saucepan and add veal mixture, cook, stirring often, for 10-15 minutes or until veal is cooked.

3. Spoon an equal amount of veal mixture onto each lettuce leaf. Serve immediately garnished with shallots.

EXCHANGES PER SERVING:
Protein 2
Vegetable ½
110 Kilojoules Optional Exchange

San Choy Bow, one serving pictured;
Fried Rice (page 36).

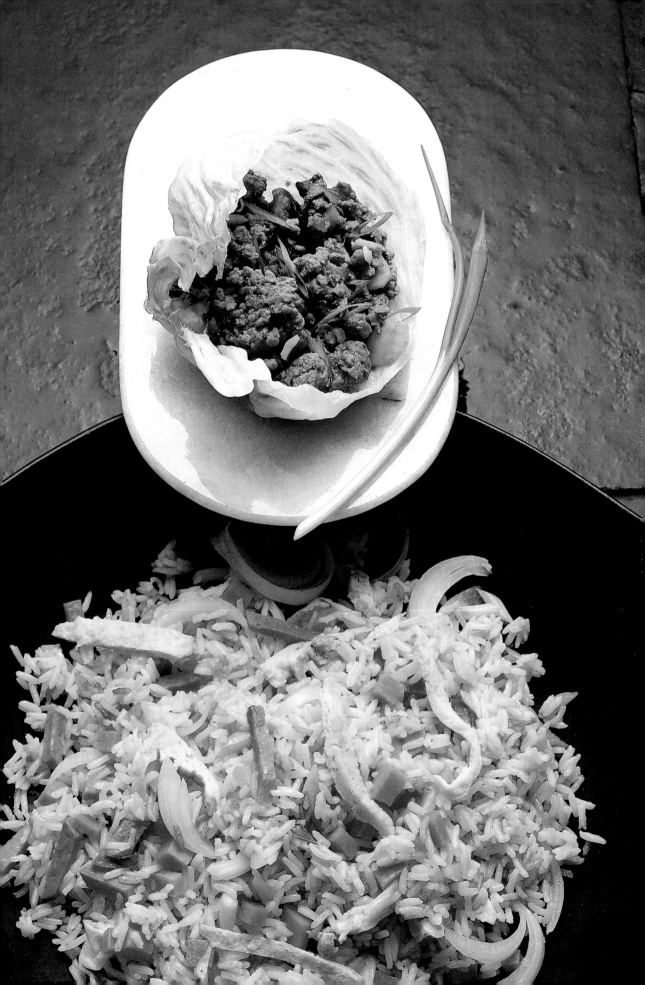

FRIED RICE

SERVES 2

This dish, pictured previous page, is a wonderful way to use up leftover rice.

2 teaspoons vegetable oil
1 egg, lightly beaten
1½ tablespoons finely chopped onion
½ garlic clove, crushed
60g leg ham, cut in thin strips
¼ cup diced carrot
1½ tablespoons frozen peas, thawed
1 cup cooked long grain rice
1½ tablespoons thinly sliced shallots
2 teaspoons soy sauce

1. Heat 1 teaspoon oil in wok, pour in egg and cook 3-5 minutes or until lightly browned, turning once. Remove egg from wok, roll up and slice thinly, set aside.

2. Heat remaining 1 teaspoon oil in wok, add onion and garlic and sauté for 2 minutes. Add ham, carrot and peas and sauté for 4 minutes.

3. Stir in remaining ingredients, except egg and toss until rice is heated through. Remove wok from heat, stir in sliced egg. Serve immediately.

EXCHANGES PER SERVING:

Protein 1½
Bread 1
Vegetable ½
Fat 1
20 Kilojoules Optional Exchange

SWEET AND SOUR PORK

—— SERVES 2 ——

Serve this dish with boiled rice to make a complete meal.

For the pork balls
278g minced pork
1 clove garlic, crushed
pinch rosemary
pinch each salt and pepper
For the sauce
1½ tablespoons cider vinegar
2 tablespoons soy sauce
3 teaspoons cornflour
3 teaspoons tomato sauce
½ medium green or red capsicum or a mixture of both, seeded and finely chopped
100g fresh pineapple, cored and chopped
1 tablespoon chopped shallots
1 vegetable stock cube, dissolved in ¾ cup water

1. Mix the pork and seasonings together, shape into eight balls, grill on rack in grilling pan until the fat stops dripping, 5-8 minutes, turning from time to time.

2. Blend the vinegar, soy sauce, cornflour and tomato sauce. Stir in the capsicum, pineapple, shallots and stock.

3. Bring to the boil, stirring all the time, reduce the heat, cover and simmer for 5-6 minutes.

4. Add the pork balls, cover and simmer for a further 5-10 minutes.

EXCHANGES PER SERVING:
Protein 3½
Vegetable ½
Fruit ½
140 Kilojoules Optional Exchange

SAVORY CASSEROLE

SERVES 2

An easy dish where fish or chicken can be substituted for the ham.

1 tablespoon polyunsaturated margarine
1 tablespoon plain flour
½ cup skim milk
1½ tablespoons tomato sauce
½ teaspoon each Worcestershire sauce and French mustard
¼ teaspoon salt
200g cooked peeled potatoes, sliced
75g finely chopped ham
30g grated tasty cheese
½ hard-cooked egg, crumbled

1. Grease a small ovenproof dish with 1 teaspoon of the margarine. Heat remaining margarine in saucepan, add flour, cook, stirring constantly for 1 minute. Remove from heat, gradually stir in milk.

2. Return to heat, cook, stirring constantly until sauce boils and thickens. Remove from heat, stir in the tomato sauce, Worcestershire sauce, mustard and salt.

3. Place alternate layers of potato, ham and sauce in prepared dish, ending with a layer of decoratively arranged potato. Sprinkle with remaining in gredients.

4. Bake at 180°C for 20-30 minutes or until heated through and cheese has melted.

EXCHANGES PER SERVING:
Protein 2
Bread 1
Fat 2
Milk ¼
175 Kilojoules Optional Exchange

Savory Casserole and Herbed Zucchini (page 80).

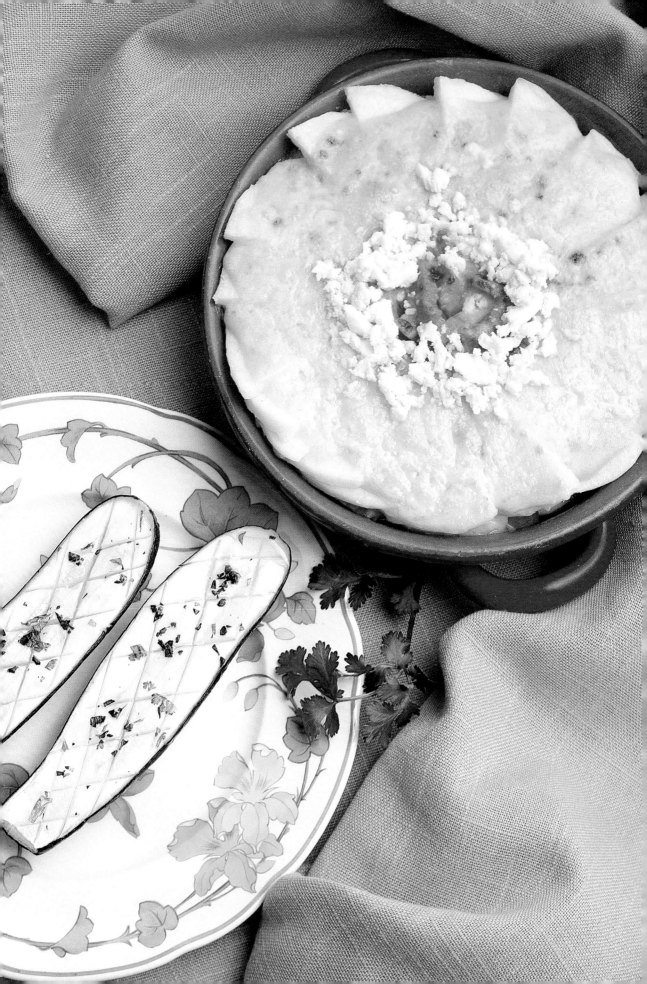

HAM STEAK WITH ORANGE AND APRICOT SAUCE

SERVES 2

The combination of oranges and apricots complements the flavor of the ham steaks.

1 cup orange juice (no sugar added)
6 dried apricot halves, chopped
¼ cup water
2 teaspoons cornflour
lemon juice to taste
2x120g ham steaks
sprigs of watercress for garnish

1. Pour the orange juice into a bowl, add the chopped apricots and leave to soak for about 4 hours or overnight.

2. Blend water and cornflour to make a paste and stir into the orange juice mixture. Bring to the boil in a saucepan, stirring all the time, reduce the heat and simmer for 2 minutes. Add lemon juice to taste.

3. While the sauce is being made, grill the ham steaks for about 8 minutes, turning once.

4. Serve the ham steaks on warm serving plates with the sauce poured over. Garnish with sprigs of watercress.

EXCHANGES PER SERVING:
Protein 4
Fruit 1½
50 Kilojoules Optional Exchange

CORNED BEEF POTATOES

SERVES 2

If you are using the oven at any temperature between 180°-200°C this is a simple snack to make. Just wash the potato, prick through the skin and bake for about an hour. If you own a microwave it is possible to cook the potato in a few minutes. Serve with a crisp green or mixed salad.

200g hot baked potato
90g corned silverside, cooked and chopped
1 tablespoon chopped shallots
1 egg, beaten
salt and pepper

1. Cut the cooked potato in half lengthwise. Carefully scoop out the potato pulp, leaving the skin intact.

2. Mash the corned silverside in a bowl. Add the potato pulp and shallots and mash once again.

3. Gradually add the beaten egg. Season the filling well.

4. Spoon the stuffing back into the potato skins and reheat under a moderate grill for 5-6 minutes until the stuffing is piping hot and browning on top.

EXCHANGES PER SERVING:
Protein 2
Bread 1

LAMB WITH FRUIT SAUCE

SERVES 2

The combination of cranberries, orange juice and redcurrant jelly complements the flavor of lamb. Don't be tempted to add more sugar to the sauce; there is sufficient in the redcurrant jelly to sweeten but still leave a slightly tart flavor.

2 x 150g lamb chump chops
For the sauce
½ cup frozen cranberries, thawed
¼ cup fresh orange juice
1½ tablespoons redcurrant jelly
1 teaspoon water
½ teaspoon arrowroot

1. Grill the lamb chops on a rack in grilling pan while making the sauce.

2. Place the cranberries and orange juice in a small saucepan, simmer gently for about 5 minutes until the cranberries start popping. Add the redcurrant jelly and stir until dissolved.

3. Blend water and arrowroot to make a paste, stir into the cranberries and bring to the boil, stirring all the time. Boil for 1 minute.

4. Serve the lamb chops on warm serving plates with the fruit sauce.

EXCHANGES PER SERVING:
Protein 3
Fruit ½
215 Kilojoules Optional Exchange

Lamb with Fruit Sauce, one serving pictured, with baby corn and snow peas.

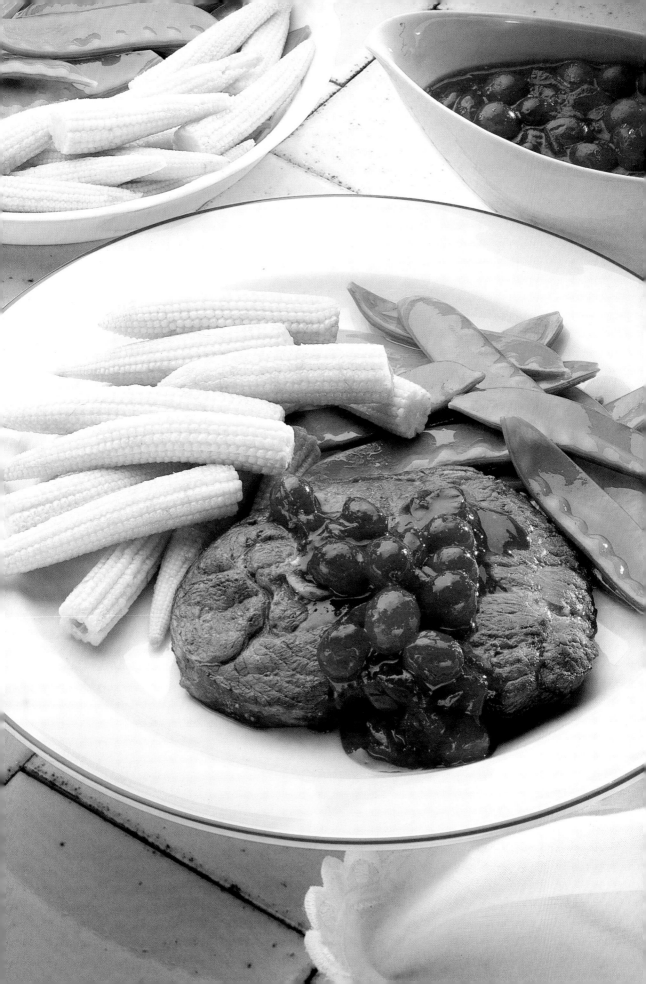

LAMB KEBABS

SERVES 2

These spicy kebabs are delicious served with boiled rice and a crisp green salad.

300g minced lamb
1½ tablespoons finely chopped onion
3 teaspoons each chopped fresh parsley and mint
¼ teaspoon each ground cumin, marjoram, salt and pepper
2 teaspoons olive oil
1 teaspoon lemon juice
½ garlic clove, crushed
¼ teaspoon paprika

1. Mix lamb, onion, herbs and seasonings together. Shape into four equal sausages, press each onto a metal skewer.

2. Combine remaining ingredients in a small bowl and brush oil mixture over kebabs.

3. Preheat grill. Place the kebabs on rack in grilling pan and cook for 10-12 minutes, turning once, or until kebabs are browned on all sides.

EXCHANGES PER SERVING:

Protein 4
Vegetable ⅛
170 Kilojoules Optional Exchange

APRICOT GLAZED LAMB

SERVES 2

This tasty lamb meal is rich in flavor but only takes minutes to make.

3 teaspoons apricot jam
1 teaspoon each French mustard, honey and soy sauce
½ garlic clove, crushed
2x150g lamb chump chops

1. Mix jam, mustard, honey, soy sauce and garlic in a small bowl.

2. Preheat grill. Place the lamb chops on rack in grilling pan and cook for 2 minutes, then brush chops with half of the apricot mixture and grill 5-7 minutes.

3. Turn chops over and grill for 2 minutes before brushing with remaining apricot mixture. Grill a further 5-7 minutes or until done to taste.

EXCHANGES PER SERVING:
Protein 3
150 Kilojoules Optional Exchange

SHEPHERD'S PIE

SERVES 2

You can also use lamb for this dish but remember to precook it in the usual way.

2 teaspoons vegetable oil
300g minced veal
½ cup thinly sliced carrot
½ cup canned tomatoes, chopped, with liquid
¼ cup diced celery
¼ cup chopped onion
1½ tablespoons tomato paste
1 teaspoon chopped fresh thyme
½ beef stock cube, dissolved in ¼ cup water
300g cooked peeled potato, hot
¼ cup skim milk
pinch each pepper and garlic salt
thyme sprig for garnish

1. Heat oil, add the veal and stir-fry for 5 minutes or until browned. Stir in carrot, canned tomato, celery, onion, tomato paste, thyme and stock. Reduce heat, cover and cook, stirring often for 15 minutes.

2. Meanwhile place potato, milk, pepper and garlic salt in a bowl and mash until smooth.

3. Place veal mixture into a casserole dish and arrange mashed potato decoratively over veal mixture and grill for 2-3 minutes until the potato is golden brown. Serve garnished with thyme sprig.

EXCHANGES PER SERVING:
Protein 4
Bread 1½
Vegetable 1¾
Fat 1
60 Kilojoules Optional Exchange

Shepherd's Pie, pictured at start of Step 3 in method.

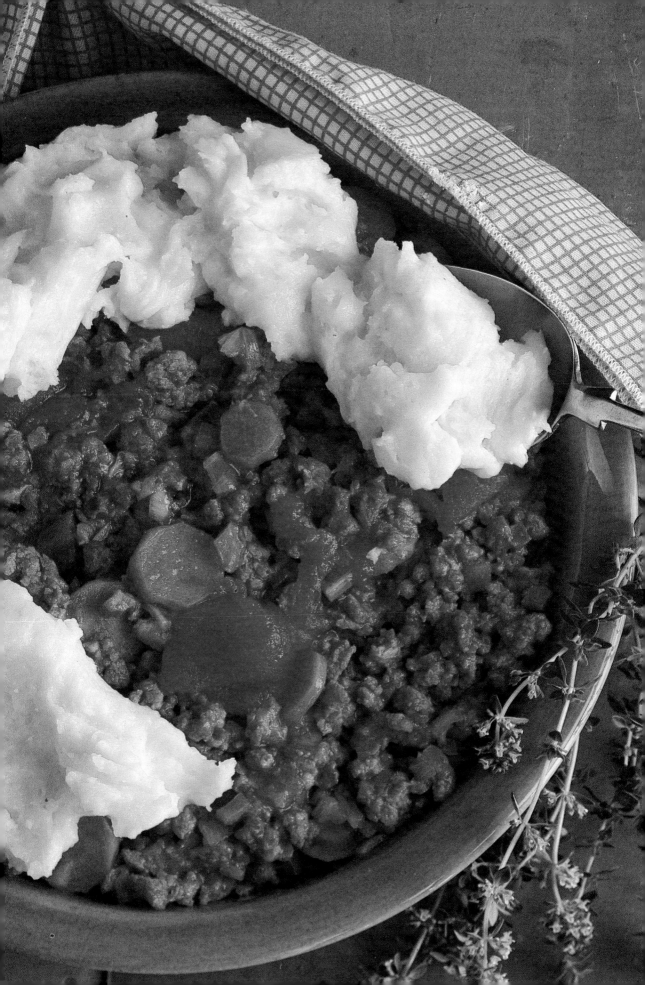

VEAL STEAK WITH LEEK AND MUSHROOM SAUCE

—— SERVES 2 ——

This recipe is easy to make and ideal for a special occasion. Serve with freshly cooked vegetables such as snow peas or green beans and carrots.

2 x 120g veal steaks
1 teaspoon lemon juice
For the sauce
1 teaspoon polyunsaturated margarine
1 small leek, thinly sliced
1 cup button mushrooms, sliced
1½ tablespoons cream
2 teaspoons chopped parsley
squeeze of lemon juice
salt and pepper
lemon wedges to garnish

1. Place the veal steaks on a grill rack in grilling pan, sprinkle over ½ teaspoon of the lemon juice and grill under a moderate heat for about 4 minutes. Turn steaks, sprinkle over remaining ½ teaspoon lemon juice and grill for a further 4-5 minutes.

2. Meanwhile, make the sauce. Heat the margarine, add the leek and stir-fry for 3 minutes. Add the mushrooms and continue stir-frying for 2-3 minutes.

3. Stir the cream and parsley into the sauce. Season to taste with squeeze of lemon juice, salt and pepper. Reheat, stirring all the time.

4. Serve the veal steaks on warm serving plates with the sauce poured over and garnished with lemon wedges.

EXCHANGES PER SERVING:
Protein 3
Vegetable 2
Fat ½
200 Kilojoules Optional Exchange

CHICKEN CASSEROLE

If yellow capsicum isn't available, use extra red and green so the casserole remains colorful.

2 x 270g chicken legs
2 teaspoons polyunsaturated margarine
1 medium onion, chopped
½ medium red capsicum, seeded and sliced
½ medium green capsicum, seeded and sliced
½ medium yellow capsicum, seeded and sliced
1 tablespoon plain flour
¼ teaspoon paprika
1 chicken stock cube, dissolved in 1 cup water
salt and pepper

1. Remove the skin from the chicken legs.

2. Melt the margarine in a heatproof casserole dish. Turn the chicken legs in the hot fat to lightly brown. Remove from the dish.

3. Add the onion and capsicum and stir-fry for 3-4 minutes over a moderate heat.

4. Stir in the flour and paprika and gradually blend in the stock. Bring to the boil, stirring all the time. Season to taste with salt and pepper. Add the chicken and cover the casserole.

5. Bake at 180°C for about 35 minutes.

EXCHANGES PER SERVING:
Protein 3
Vegetable 2½
Fat 1
125 Kilojoules Optional Exchange

LIVER STIR-UP

SERVES 2

This family favorite can be adapted to use up any vegetables from the garden or vegetable basket. Serve with pasta.

1½ tablespoons plain flour

salt and pepper

150g lamb's fry, thinly sliced

2 teaspoons vegetable oil

1 medium onion, thinly sliced

1 medium carrot, cut into thin strips

1 medium zucchini, sliced

1 x 40g rasher Danish-style bacon, very lean, grilled and cut into strips

¼ vegetable or chicken stock cube, dissolved in ¼ cup water

⅓ cup low-fat natural yoghurt

---

1. Season the flour with salt and pepper. Turn liver in the seasoned flour, put to one side.

2. Heat the oil in a medium saucepan, add the onion and sauté 2-3 minutes.

3. Add the liver and stir-fry for 2 minutes until brown.

4. Stir in the carrot, zucchini, bacon and stock. Bring to the boil, reduce the heat, cover and simmer for 5 minutes.

5. Remove from the heat, stir in the yoghurt and serve.

EXCHANGES PER SERVING:
Protein 2½
Vegetable 3
Fat 1
Milk ¼
185 Kilojoules Optional Exchange

Liver Stir-up, served with pasta.

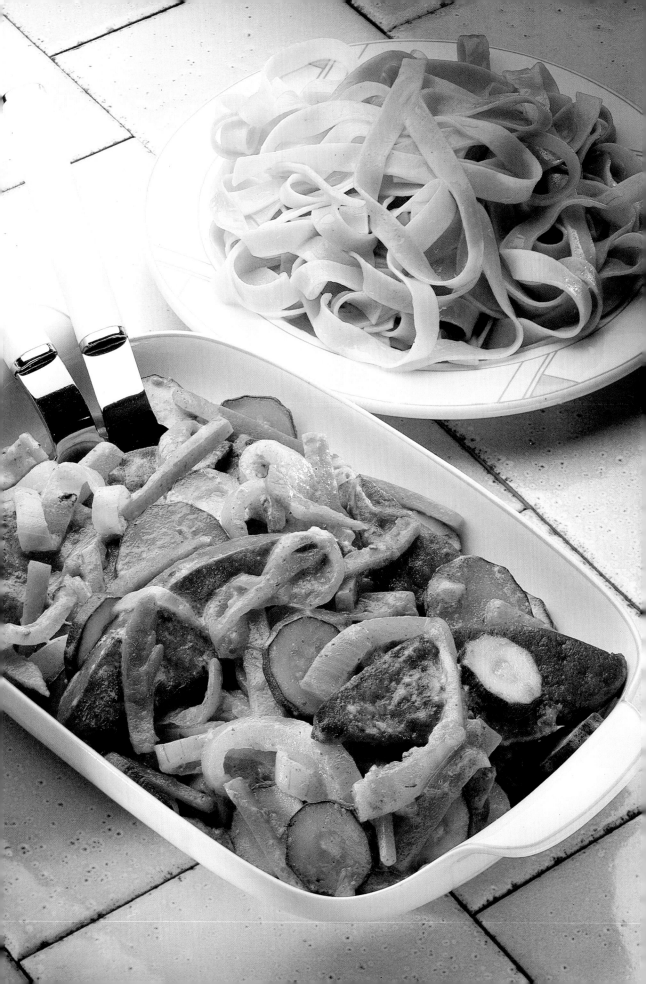

SPICY CHICKEN BURGER

A quick and easy meal for one, great cooked on the barbecue.

---

1 x 120g chicken thigh fillet

½ teaspoon chicken seasoning

1x60g hamburger bun, halved and toasted

½ medium tomato, sliced

¼ cup shredded lettuce

---

1. Place chicken fillet on a grill rack, sprinkle over half of the chicken seasoning and grill under a moderate heat for about 6 minutes. Turn over and sprinkle the remaining chicken seasoning over and grill for a further 6-8 minutes.

2. Place chicken on bottom half of bun and top with tomato slices and lettuce. Cover with top half of bun.

EXCHANGES PER SERVING:
Protein 3
Bread 2
Vegetable 1½

CURRIED CHICKEN WITH BROCCOLI

--- SERVES 2 ---

A tasty way to use up leftover chicken for that meal in a hurry.

300g broccoli
For the sauce
2 teaspoons polyunsaturated margarine
1½ tablespoons chopped onion
1 teaspoon curry powder
1 tablespoon plain flour
½ cup evaporated skim milk
½ chicken stock cube, dissolved in ¼ cup water
pinch pepper
240g boned cooked chicken breast, cut into 4 slices

1. Cut the broccoli into even-sized pieces. Boil in salted water until just cooked but still crisp, 8-10 minutes.

2. While broccoli is boiling, make the curry sauce. Melt margarine over a medium heat, add onion and curry powder and cook 1 minute. Add flour and stir over heat for a further minute.

3. Gradually whisk in the evaporated milk, chicken stock and pepper.

4. Bring the sauce to the boil, stirring all the time, reduce heat and simmer for about 3 minutes. Add chicken slices and turn to coat with sauce, cook until heated through.

5. Arrange hot broccoli on a serving plate and top with chicken and sauce.

EXCHANGES PER SERVING:
Protein 4
Vegetable 2¾
Fat 1
Milk ½
115 Kilojoules Optional Exchange

VEAL ROAST

SERVES 4

An easy weekend roast, great for when friends come to visit.

⅓ cup dry white wine
1½ tablespoons lemon juice
¼ teaspoon mustard powder
¼ teaspoon crushed garlic
pinch freshly ground black pepper
600g boned, rolled and tied veal roast
parsley to garnish

1. Combine all ingredients except veal in a bowl. Pour over the veal, cover and refrigerate, several hours or overnight, turning frequently.

2. Preheat oven to 160°C. Place veal in roasting pan and place meat thermometer into thickest part of veal.

3. Bake for about 35 minutes or until meat thermometer registers 75°C, basting often with marinade. Serve garnished with parsley.

EXCHANGES PER SERVING:
Protein 4
105 Kilojoules Optional Exchange

Veal Roast and Nutty Damper (page 113).

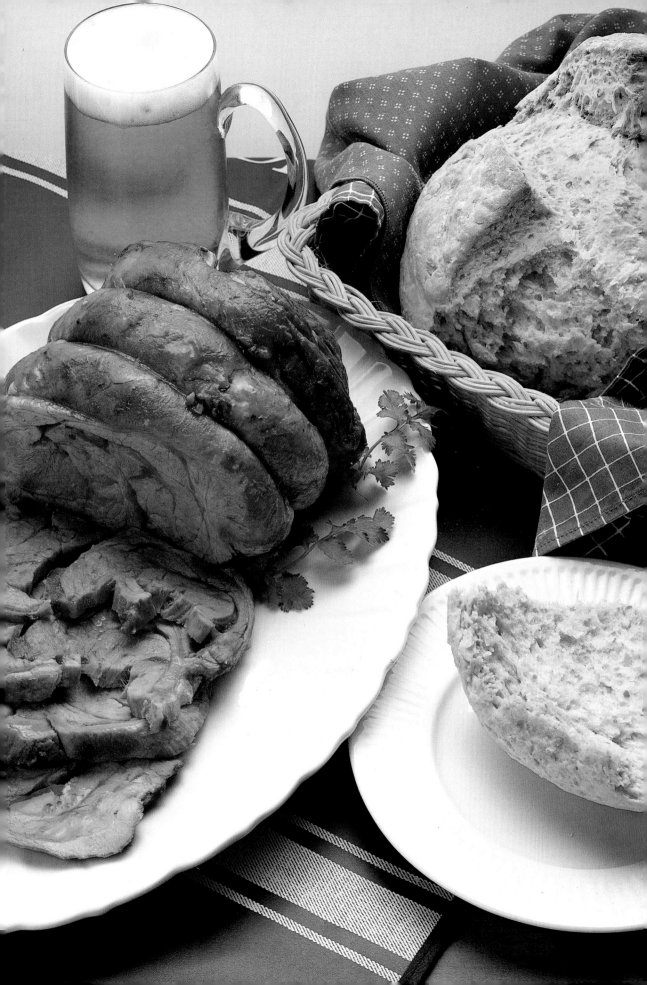

CHICKEN IN WINE SAUCE

SERVES 2

Serve this flavorsome chicken dish with a green salad or crisp vegetables.

300g chicken thigh fillets
⅛ teaspoon paprika
pinch freshly ground pepper
For the sauce
2 teaspoons polyunsaturated margarine
¼ cup finely chopped mushrooms
1 tablespoon finely chopped onion
¼ teaspoon crushed garlic
2 teaspoons plain flour
pinch each salt and pepper
1 tablespoon dry red wine
¼ chicken stock cube, dissolved in ¼ cup water

1. Sprinkle chicken evenly with paprika and pepper. In a medium pan that has been sprayed with non-stick cooking spray cook chicken for about 7 minutes, turning once. Place chicken in a medium casserole dish.

2. In same pan melt margarine, add mushrooms, onion and garlic and stir-fry for 4 minutes. Stir in flour, salt and pepper and cook, stirring constantly for 3 minutes.

3. Preheat oven to 180°C. Whisk in wine and stock and simmer for 10 minutes, stirring often. Pour sauce over chicken, stir and cover.

4. Bake for about 20 minutes.

EXCHANGES PER SERVING:
Protein 4
Vegetable ¼
Fat 1
105 Kilojoules Optional Exchange

SEAFOOD

The harvest from the sea produces a wide and interesting variety of foods, from exotic shellfish to plain white fish which contains very little fat. Preparation of seafood is only limited by your imagination. Whether you prepare your seafood under the griller, bake, steam or cook it in foil, there is a recipe to suit you.

OYSTER MORNAY

SERVES 2

This recipe makes an appetising starter to any dinner party.

1 tablespoon polyunsaturated margarine
1 tablespoon plain flour
½ cup skim milk
1 teaspoon lemon juice
½ teaspoon Worcestershire sauce
6 medium oysters in shells
1 teaspoon vegetable oil
1 tablespoon grated cheese
2 teaspoons dried breadcrumbs
½ teaspoon chopped fresh parsley

1. Melt margarine, add flour, cook, stirring constantly for 1 minute. Gradually whisk in milk.

2. Bring the sauce to the boil, stirring continually, reduce heat and simmer for about 3 minutes. Stir in the lemon juice and Worcestershire sauce.

3. Remove oysters from shells and grease shells with oil. Place a teaspoon of the sauce into each shell, replace oysters, top with remaining sauce.

4. Preheat oven to 180°C. Mix remaining ingredients and sprinkle over oysters.

5. Bake for 10-15 minutes or until cheese has melted and is bubbling.

EXCHANGES PER SERVING:
Protein 1
Fat 2½
Milk ¼
250 Kilojoules Optional Exchange

Oyster Mornay and Avocado Salad (page 92).

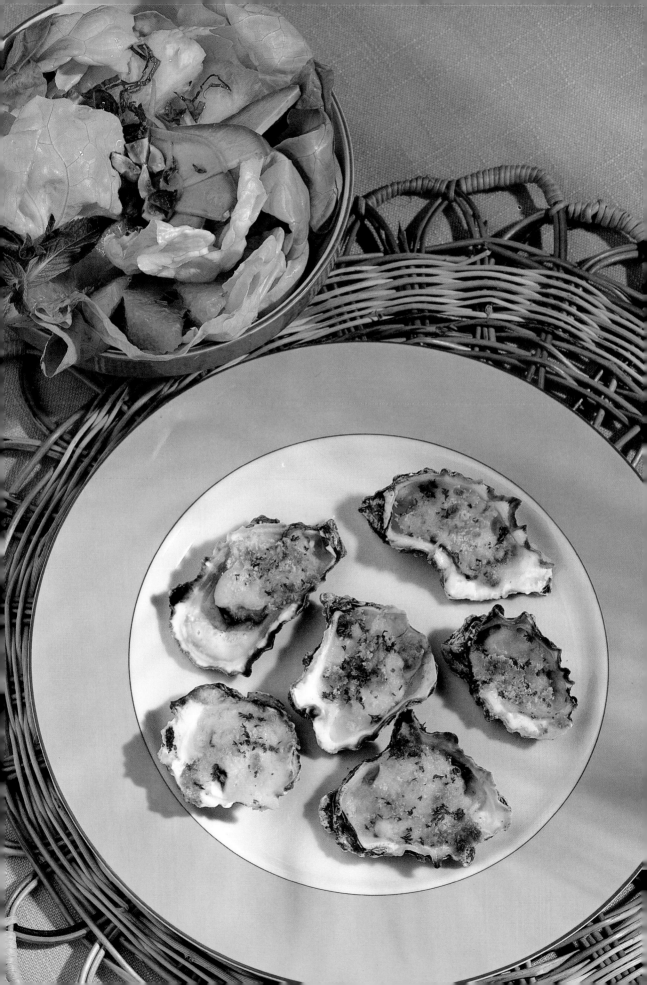

FISH AND SCALLOP KEBABS

SERVES 2

Baste these kebabs frequently during cooking to prevent them drying out. Serve with plain boiled rice.

For the kebabs
120g jewfish fillet
120g Tasmanian scallops
$\frac{1}{2}$ medium green capsicum, seeded
3 button mushrooms, halved
2 shallots, each cut into four pieces
4 cherry tomatoes
For the marinade
3 teaspoons olive or vegetable oil
$1\frac{1}{2}$ tablespoons lemon juice
$\frac{1}{2}$ teaspoon marjoram
$\frac{1}{2}$ teaspoon thyme
salt and pepper

1. Cut the jewfish into four cubes. Place the fish and scallops into a dish.

2. Whisk together all the marinade ingredients, pour over the fish and leave to marinate 1-2 hours.

3. Cut the green capsicum into cubes, plunge into boiling water, boil for 3 minutes, drain.

4. Thread the fish, scallops, capsicum, mushrooms and shallots onto four skewers, ending with a tomato.

5. Place the kebabs under a preheated grill, cook for 5-7 minutes, turning and basting frequently with the marinade.

EXCHANGES PER SERVING:
Protein 3
Vegetable $1\frac{1}{8}$
255 Kilojoules Optional Exchange

HOT SHERRIED PRAWNS

SERVES 2

Serve this dish with boiled rice and crisp lightly cooked broccoli to make a complete meal. Don't over-cook the prawns as they shrink.

180g cooked peeled prawns
¼ cup dry or medium sherry
1 teaspoon finely chopped fresh green ginger
1 clove garlic, crushed
1 teaspoon vegetable oil
½ medium zucchini, cut in thin strips
1½ tablespoons chopped shallots
½ cup bean sprouts
salt and pepper
3 teaspoons chopped coriander

1. Place the prawns in a dish, stir in the sherry, ginger and garlic, cover and refrigerate for about 2 hours.

2. Heat the oil, add the zucchini and shallots and stir-fry for 2 minutes.

3. Pour the sherried prawns and the marinade into the zucchini mixture, add the bean sprouts and stir over a moderate heat 4-5 minutes. Season to taste and stir in the chopped coriander.

EXCHANGES PER SERVING:
Protein 3
Vegetable 1⅛
Fat ½
155 Kilojoules Optional Exchange

SMOKED SALMON ROLLS

SERVES 2

When you feel like spoiling yourself, this is the recipe to make. It can either be eaten by two for lunch or supper or it may be served to four people as an appetiser.

180g cottage cheese
2 teaspoons chopped chives
1 teaspoon lemon juice
pepper
4 x 30g thin slices smoked salmon
8 endive leaves
lemon slices to garnish

1. Mix together the cottage cheese, chives and lemon juice, season with pepper.

2. Lay the smoked salmon slices out and spread the cheese mixture over the length of each slice. Roll up Swiss roll style.

3. Arrange the endive leaves on the serving plates, transfer 2 salmon rolls to each plate and garnish with the lemon slices.

EXCHANGES PER SERVING:
Protein 3½
Vegetable ½

Smoked Salmon Rolls.

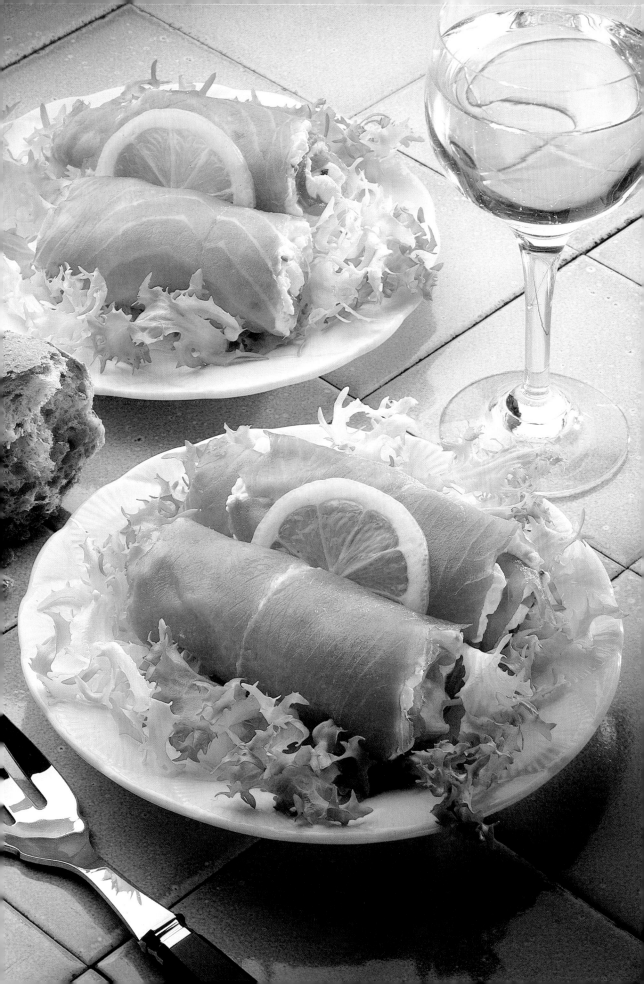

KEDGEREE

SERVES 2

This is a favorite dish. Prepare it in advance and heat it up when needed. You can adapt the recipe to incorporate other ingredients you have on hand, for example, red or green capsicum.

190g smoked haddock or cod fillets, skinned
½ cup long grain brown rice
1 hard-cooked egg, chopped
4 shallots, finely chopped
⅓ cup low-fat natural yoghurt
2 tablespoons chopped parsley
salt and pepper

1. Place the fish in a pan, cover with cold water and heat gently. Poach for about 10 minutes. Remove the fish from the water and flake with a fork.

2. Boil the rice in the poaching water following the pack instructions and adding more water if necessary, for 40 minutes.

3. Drain the rice if any liquid remains. Stir the flaked fish, egg, shallots, yoghurt and parsley into the rice and mix well. Heat gently, stirring all the time. Season well and serve.

EXCHANGES PER SERVING:

Protein 3
Bread 1½
Vegetable ¼
Milk ¼
95 Kilojoules Optional Exchange

ROLLED FLOUNDER FILLETS

SERVES 2

Serve these fillets with a selection of hot, colorful vegetables to make a filling meal.

60g cooked peeled and deveined prawns, chopped
1 slice white bread, made into crumbs
3 teaspoons chopped parsley
3 teaspoons chopped chives
3 teaspoons finely grated Parmesan cheese
2 tablespoons skim milk
salt and pepper
2x120g flounder fillets
½ teaspoon polyunsaturated margarine
lemon wedges to serve

1. Mix together the prawns, breadcrumbs, herbs and cheese. Add milk to bind, and season with salt and pepper.

2. Spread half of the stuffing along one side of each of the fillets, roll up and secure with cocktail sticks.

3. Use half of the margarine to grease a small ovenproof dish just large enough to hold the fillets, dot the remaining margarine on top of the flounder and cover loosely with foil.

4. Bake at 180°C for 20 minutes. Serve with lemon wedges.

EXCHANGES PER SERVING:

Protein 4
Bread ½
150 Kilojoules Optional Exchange

PAELLA

SERVES 2

This traditional Spanish dish is a combination of various seafood and meat. If preferred, use long grain brown rice but increase the boiling water by about ¼ cup.

2 teaspoons vegetable or olive oil	salt and pepper
1 medium onion, chopped	90g unpeeled prawns
1 medium red capsicum, seeded and chopped	60g cooked peeled and deveined prawns
1 clove garlic, finely chopped	60g cooked chicken, diced
2 medium tomatoes, peeled and chopped	4 medium mussels, steamed
1 cup water	40g scallops
½ cup long grain rice	2 teaspoons chopped parsley
juice of ½ a lemon	lemon wedges and parsley sprigs to garnish
pinch of powdered saffron	

1. Heat the oil in a saucepan, add the onion, red capsicum and garlic, stir-fry 3-4 minutes.

2. Stir in the chopped tomatoes, water, rice, lemon juice and saffron, season with salt and pepper. Bring to the boil, stirring all the time, cover, reduce the heat and simmer for 12 minutes.

3. Add the prawns, chicken, mussels and scallops and stir over a moderate heat for a few minutes until the rice and scallops are cooked, the liquid absorbed, and the chicken and prawns heated through.

4. Transfer to a serving dish, sprinkle with parsley and garnish with lemon wedges and parsley sprigs.

EXCHANGES PER SERVING:
Protein 4
Bread 1½
Vegetable 4
Fat 1
50 Kilojoules Optional Exchange

Paella.

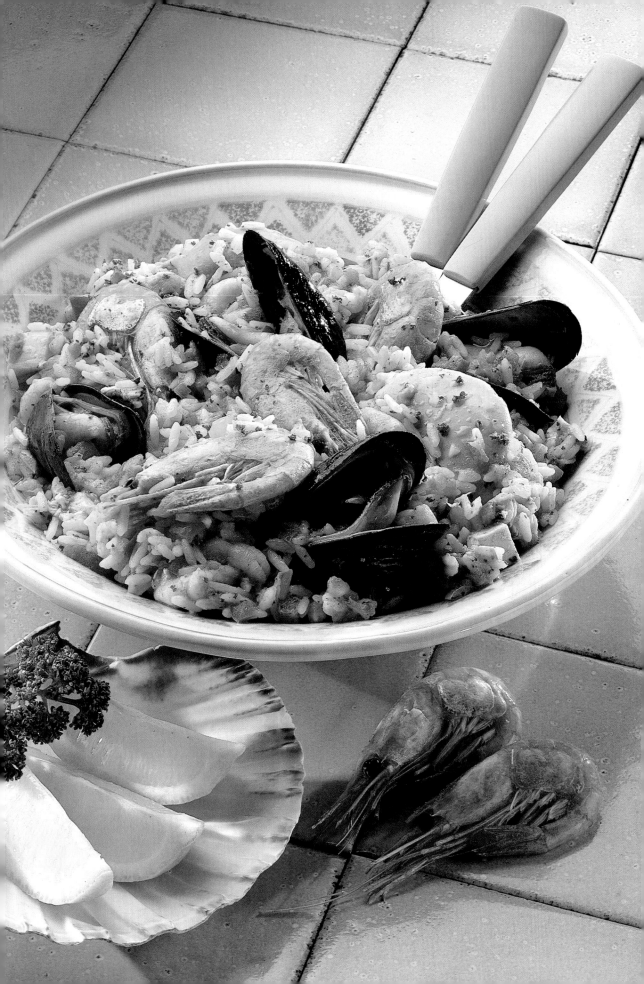

CHEESE-TOPPED COD

SERVES 2

This simple dish can be altered in a number of ways: either use a different fish, such as haddock or flounder, or replace the fennel with parsley or chervil.

2 x 120g cod fillets
½ teaspoon polyunsaturated margarine
30g cheese, grated
1 teaspoon chopped fennel
1 medium tomato, sliced

1. Dot the skin-side of the fish fillets with half of the margarine, grill for 4 minutes under a moderate heat.

2. Turn the fillets over, dot with remaining margarine and grill for 2 minutes.

3. Sprinkle the cheese and fennel over the fillets, place half of the tomato slices over each fillet and return to the grill for a further 2-3 minutes until the cheese has melted and is bubbling.

EXCHANGES PER SERVING:
Protein 3½
Vegetable 1
45 Kilojoules Optional Exchange

SMOTHERED FISH

SERVES 2

The combination of tomatoes, herbs and olives with fish makes an interesting main course. For a change, substitute the oregano with 1-2 teaspoons freshly chopped chervil

1 teaspoon olive oil
270g whiting fillets
1 medium onion, thinly sliced
½ medium green capsicum, seeded and cut into strips
1 clove garlic, finely chopped
¼ teaspoon oregano
¼ teaspoon basil
pinch each salt and pepper
4 black olives, stoned and halved
1 medium tomato blanched, peeled and sliced

1. Use ¼ teaspoon of the oil to brush the base of an ovenproof dish, just long enough to hold the whiting, and about 5cm deep. Place the whiting in the dish.

2. Heat the remaining oil in a saucepan, add the onion, green capsicum and garlic and stir-fry about 4 minutes.

3. Spread the onion, green capsicum and garlic on top of the whiting, sprinkle with the herbs and salt and pepper. Add the olives.

4. Lay the tomato slices over the top, sprinkle with a little more salt and pepper, cover with foil and bake at 180°C for 35 minutes.

EXCHANGES PER SERVING:
Protein 3½
Vegetable 2½
Fat ½
20 Kilojoules Optional Exchange

STEAMED FISH WITH VEGETABLES

———————————————— SERVES 2 ————————————————

This simple dish requires only one saucepan and takes about 10-15 minutes to cook. Make your choice from cod, haddock or flounder.

2 teaspoons polyunsaturated margarine
1 medium leek, thinly sliced
1 medium carrot, thinly sliced
1 medium zucchini, thinly sliced
1 tablespoon chopped chervil
$\frac{1}{4}$ vegetable stock cube, dissolved in $\frac{1}{3}$ cup water
2x150g cod, haddock or flounder fillets
salt and pepper
2 teaspoons chopped parsley to garnish

1. Melt the margarine in a large saucepan, add the leek and stir-fry for 1 minute. Add the carrot, zucchini, chervil and stock. Bring to the boil.

2. Place the fillets of fish on the top of the vegetables, season with salt and pepper. Tightly cover the saucepan, reduce the heat and cook gently for 10-15 minutes, until the fish is just cooked. Garnish with chopped parsley.

EXCHANGES PER SERVING:
Protein 4
Vegetable 2¼
Fat 1
5 Kilojoules Optional Exchange

Steamed Fish with Vegetables.

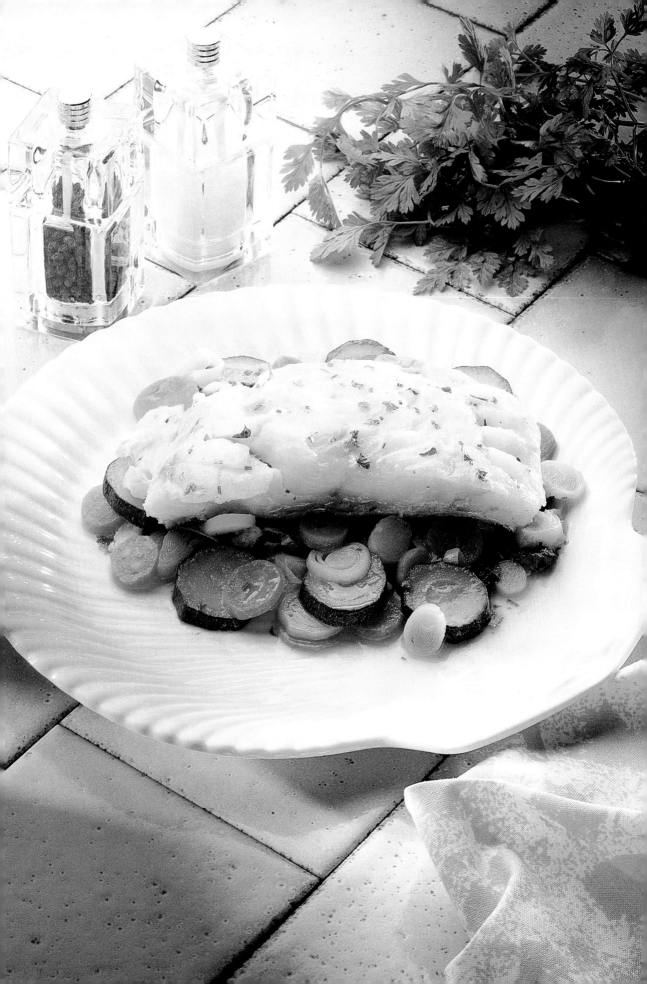

PACKAGED SALMON

SERVES 2

It's doubtful a recipe could be much simpler to prepare than this one, yet it retains the texture of the salmon, looks attractive and tastes delicious.

¼ teaspoon polyunsaturated margarine
2x180g salmon steaks
2 teaspoons chopped chervil
2 thin slices lemon
salt and pepper

1. With the margarine lightly grease a piece of foil large enough to hold the salmon steaks.

2. Preheat oven to 190°C. Place the salmon steaks on the greased foil, sprinkle with the chervil and place the lemon slices on top. Season with salt and pepper.

3. Fold the foil over to form a parcel. Bake for 20 minutes.

EXCHANGES PER SERVING:
Protein 4
20 Kilojoules Optional Exchange

STUFFED TROUT

SERVES 2

It's well worth looking out for small trout for this dish. They are easy to prepare and can be just sprinkled with lemon juice and a few chopped herbs, such as chervil or parsley, wrapped in foil and baked or stuffed as described below.

2 teaspoons polyunsaturated margarine
½ small onion, finely chopped
½ cup mushrooms, chopped
1 slice white bread, made into crumbs
1½ tablespoons chopped parsley
3 teaspoons lemon juice
1 egg, beaten
salt and pepper
2x205g trout, cleaned with heads on
lemon wedges to serve
sprigs of parsley to garnish

1. Use ½ teaspoon of the margarine to grease a piece of foil large enough to hold the trout.

2. Heat the remaining margarine in a saucepan, add the onion and stir-fry 3-4 minutes, add the mushrooms and cook for a further 1-2 minutes.

3. Mix the breadcrumbs, parsley and lemon juice into the mixture, bind together with the beaten egg and season with salt and pepper.

4. Preheat oven to 190°C. Wash the trout and dab dry with paper towel. Divide the stuffing between the two fish. Wrap loosely in foil and bake for 20 minutes. The eyes of the trout will turn white when cooked.

5. Serve with lemon wedges and garnish with sprigs of parsley.

EXCHANGES PER SERVING:
Protein 4
Bread ½
Vegetable ¾
Fat 1

BAKED SNAPPER

A colorful fish dish guaranteed to impress your guests.

1 teaspoon vegetable oil
½ cup chopped onion
1 garlic clove, crushed
1½ cups canned tomatoes, chopped
¼ cup chopped green capsicum
1 tablespoon lemon juice
1 teaspoon oregano
⅛ teaspoon black pepper
¼ teaspoon salt
1080g whole snapper, scaled and cleaned

1. Heat oil in medium saucepan, add onion and half the garlic, cook, stirring constantly for 2 minutes. Add tomatoes, capsicum, lemon juice, oregano and pepper, bring to the boil, reduce heat and simmer for 10 minutes, stirring often.

2. Meanwhile mix remaining garlic with salt and rub into cavity of fish. Allow to stand for 10 minutes.

3. Preheat oven to 180°C. Spread ¼ cup tomato mixture inside fish cavity and wrap fish in foil that has been sprayed with non-stick cooking spray.

4. Bake for about 35 minutes or until fish flakes easily when tested with a fork.

5. Serve fish with remaining tomato mixture.

EXCHANGES PER SERVING:
Protein 4
Vegetable ¾
30 Kilojoules Optional Exchange

Baked Snapper and Mediterranean Salad (page 89).

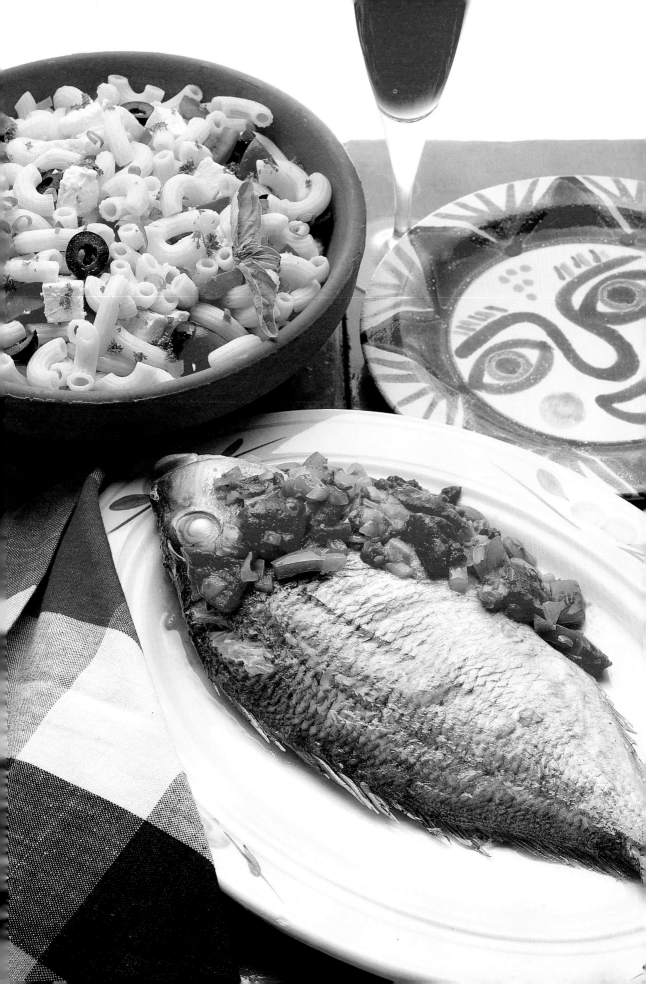

COD WITH PARSLEY SAUCE

—— SERVES 2 ——

Serve this recipe with green beans and tomatoes which have been halved, sprinkled with basil and grilled.

230g cod fillets
⅛ cup onion rings
½ bay leaf
¾ cup skim milk
salt and pepper
2 teaspoons polyunsaturated margarine
1 tablespoon plain flour
1 tablespoon chopped parsley

1. Place the cod, onion rings and bay leaf in a saucepan, pour over the milk and sprinkle with salt and pepper. Cover the pan and simmer gently for 10 minutes.

2. Melt the margarine in a separate saucepan, add the flour and remove from the heat.

3. When the fish is cooked, transfer to warm serving plates and keep warm while completing the sauce.

4. Strain the cooking liquid and gradually blend a little at a time into the margarine and flour.

5. Add the parsley and bring to the boil, stirring all the time. Boil 1-2 minutes, pour over the cod and serve.

EXCHANGES PER SERVING:
Protein 3
Vegetable ⅛
Fat 1
Milk ¼
150 Kilojoules Optional Exchange

VEGETABLES

Vegetables add variety of flavor and texture as well as supplying essential nutrients and dietary fibre. By using a wide range of different vegetables meals become increasingly appetising. When shopping for your vegetables choose good quality fresh produce.

CARROT AND ORANGE SOUP

SERVES 2

The sweetness of carrots is complemented by the tang of oranges. If you enjoy this soup, try the same combination as a salad using grated carrots and an orange juice dressing.

1 medium leek, thinly sliced
3 medium carrots, chopped
1½ vegetable stock cubes, dissolved in 1½ cups water
pinch thyme
juice of ½ a small orange
salt and pepper

1. Reserve a few slices of leek, place the remainder in a saucepan with the carrots, stock and thyme. Bring to the boil, reduce the heat, cover and simmer for 30 minutes. Allow to cool.

2. Transfer the cooked vegetables and stock to a blender or food processor and process until smooth.

3. Return the purée to the saucepan, add the orange juice and season well. Stir over a moderate heat, until heated through, pour into warm serving bowls and garnish with the reserved leek separated into rings.

EXCHANGES PER SERVING:
Vegetable 3¼
65 Kilojoules Optional Exchange

Carrot and Orange Soup.

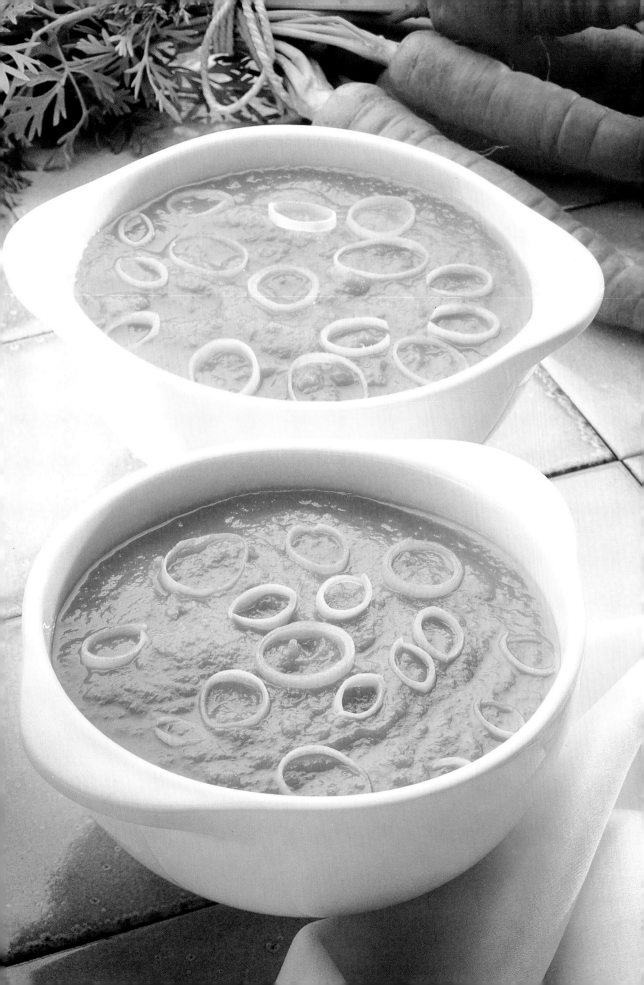

HERBED ZUCCHINI

SERVES 2

Try serving this vegetable with the Savory Casserole, both pictured on page 39.

1 medium zucchini
1 teaspoon lemon juice
½ teaspoon mixed herbs
⅛ teaspoon each salt and pepper

1. Cut zucchini in half lengthwise and score cut side of each zucchini half diagonally to make a diamond pattern.

2. Preheat oven to 190°C. Sprinkle each zucchini half with half of the lemon juice, herbs, salt and pepper. Place cut side up on baking sheet.

3. Bake for about 15 minutes or until tender. Serve immediately.

EXCHANGES PER SERVING:

Vegetable 1

VEGETABLE CURRY

SERVES 2

This recipe makes a delicious curry which can be eaten as a snack or made into a more substantial meal by adding 120g drained, cooked kidney beans. This, of course, will add 1 Protein Exchange per serving.

2 cups of mixed vegetables chosen from the following: cauliflower, turnip, pumpkin, zucchini
2 teaspoons vegetable oil
$\frac{1}{2}$ small chilli, seeded and finely chopped
1 clove garlic, finely chopped
$\frac{1}{4}$ teaspoon cumin seeds
$\frac{1}{4}$ teaspoon ground coriander
$\frac{1}{4}$ teaspoon turmeric
1 teaspoon finely chopped ginger
1 medium onion, chopped
$\frac{1}{2}$ medium okra, halved
$1\frac{1}{2}$ tablespoons tomato purée
1 vegetable stock cube, dissolved in $1\frac{1}{4}$ cups water

1. Break the cauliflower into florets, cut the turnip, pumpkin and zucchini into 2.5cm cubes.

2. Heat the oil in a saucepan. Add the chilli, garlic and spices, stir over a moderate heat for 1-2 minutes.

3. Add all the remaining ingredients, mix well and bring to the boil. Cover the saucepan and simmer for 15 minutes. Remove the saucepan lid and simmer for a further 10 minutes.

EXCHANGES PER SERVING:
Vegetable 4
Fat 1
25 Kilojoules Optional Exchange

RATATOUILLE

This colorful dish is suitable for a midday or light evening meal. It can be cooked in the oven or simmered gently on the stove for 30-40 minutes.

1 small eggplant, cubed
salt
2 teaspoons vegetable or olive oil
1 medium onion, chopped
1 medium green, red or yellow capsicum (or a mixture), seeded and sliced
1 clove garlic, finely chopped
2 medium zucchini, thickly sliced
1½ cups canned tomatoes
1 tablespoon tomato purée
½ teaspoon dried basil or 2 teaspoons chopped fresh basil
2 teaspoons chopped parsley to garnish

1. Sprinkle the eggplant with salt, leave to drain 20-30 minutes then rinse well and pat dry.

2. Heat the oil in a large heatproof casserole. Add the onion, capsicum and garlic and sauté 2-3 minutes.

3. Preheat oven to 180°C. Mix in the zucchini, tomatoes, tomato purée and basil. Stir around to break up the tomatoes.

4. Cover the casserole and bake for 45 minutes. Serve sprinkled with chopped parsley.

EXCHANGES PER SERVING:
Vegetable 7¾
Fat 1

Ratatouille

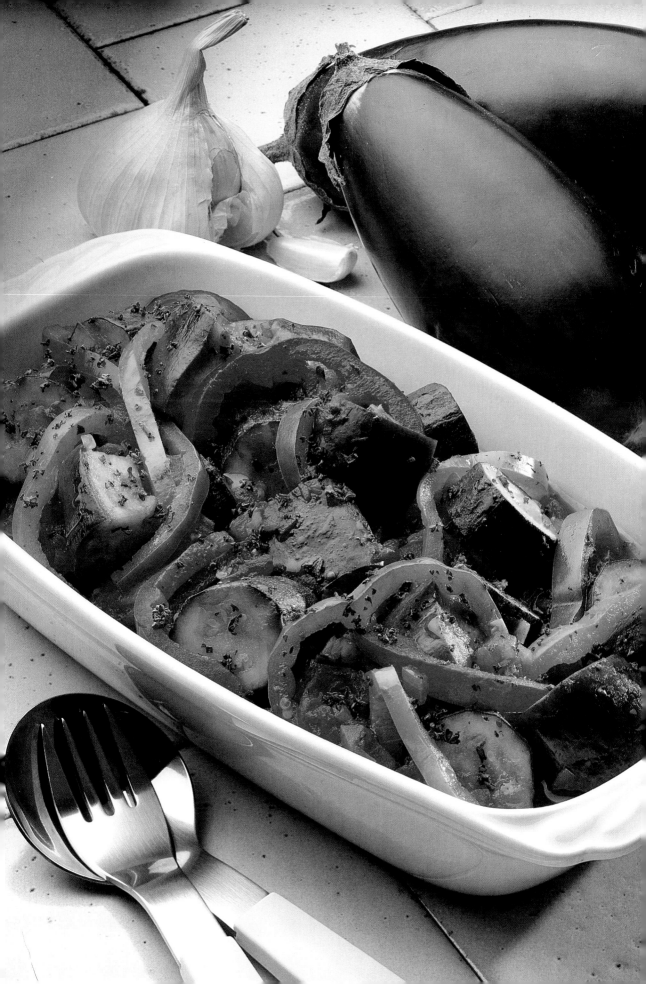

HOT SNOW PEA SALAD

SERVES 2

The peas are just topped and tailed and then everything is eaten. This method of cooking retains the flavor and crisp texture of the peas.

2 teaspoons olive oil
1 teaspoon finely chopped fresh green ginger
1 cup snow peas, topped and tailed
½ medium red capsicum, seeded and cut into thin strips
3 teaspoons red wine vinegar
salt and pepper

1. Heat the oil, add the ginger and stir-fry for 1 minute.

2. Mix in the snow peas and stir-fry for 2 minutes.

3. Add the capsicum and vinegar and cook for a further 1-2 minutes stirring all the time. Season with salt and pepper. Serve immediately.

EXCHANGES PER SERVING:
Vegetable 1½
Fat 1

CREAMY SPINACH SALAD

SERVES 2

Use only English spinach or young silverbeet leaves which are absolutely fresh for this recipe. The older leaves are far too tough and would ruin the salad.

8 English spinach leaves
1 cup shredded Chinese cabbage
1 cup button mushrooms, sliced
For the dressing
$\frac{1}{2}$ teaspoon coriander seeds
3 teaspoons cream cheese
pinch mild chilli powder
$\frac{1}{3}$ cup low-fat natural yoghurt

1. Tear or cut the spinach leaves in half. Mix together with the Chinese cabbage and mushrooms.

2. Roughly crush the coriander seeds in a small bowl using the back of a teaspoon or end of a rolling pin. Add the cream cheese and chilli powder, gradually mix in the yoghurt a tablespoon at a time.

3. Pour the dressing over the salad and toss well. Allow to stand for about an hour for the dressing flavors to be absorbed.

EXCHANGES PER SERVING:
Vegetable 2½
Milk ¼
130 Kilojoules Optional Exchange

STIR-FRIED VEGETABLES

SERVES 2

This quick recipe retains the flavor and texture of the vegetables. Sliced leeks, zucchini or celery can always be added or used to substitute for the beans and carrot.

3 teaspoons vegetable oil
1 teaspoon finely chopped green ginger
1 clove garlic, finely chopped
1 medium carrot, cut in thin strips
½ medium red capsicum, seeded and cut in strips
½ cup green beans, cut in 2.5cm pieces
½ cup bean sprouts
4 shallots, cut in thick diagonal slices
2 tablespoons water
1 tablespoon sherry
1 tablespoon tomato purée
2 teaspoons soy sauce
salt and pepper
½ teaspoon sesame seeds, toasted

1. Heat the oil in a saucepan. Add the ginger and garlic and stir-fry for 1-2 minutes. Mix in all the remaining vegetables and stir-fry for a further 3 minutes.

2. Mix the water, sherry, tomato purée and soy sauce together, pour over the vegetables and stir well.

3. Cover the saucepan and simmer for 6 minutes. Season with salt and pepper and transfer to a warm serving dish, sprinkle with sesame seeds and serve immediately.

EXCHANGES PER SERVING:
Vegetable 3
Fat 1½
75 Kilojoules Optional Exchange

Stir-fried Vegetables.

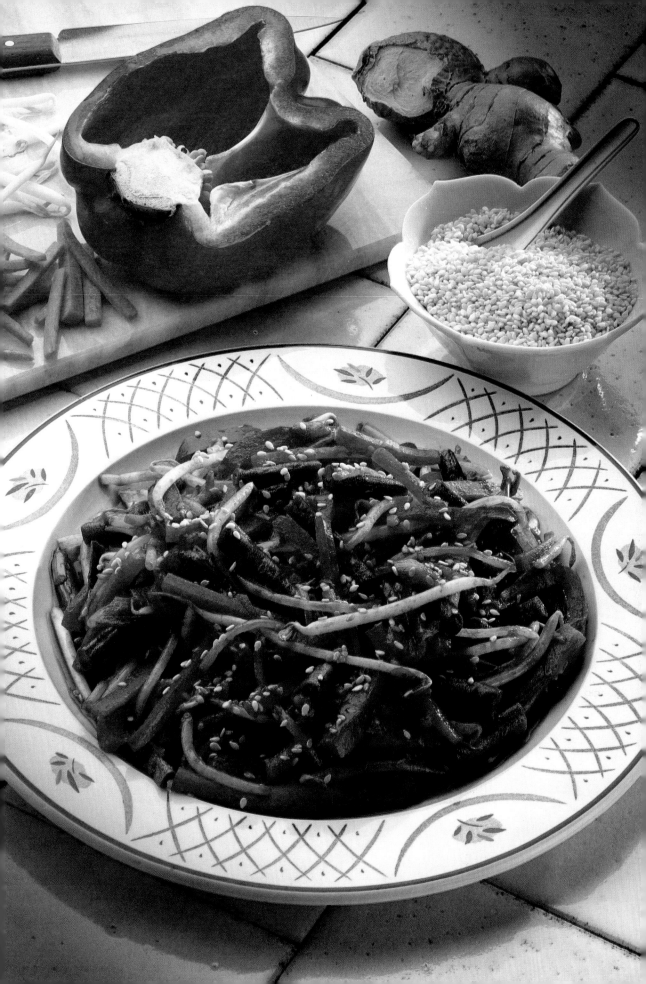

SIMPLE COLESLAW

SERVES 2

This crunchy salad is quick and simple to make. It keeps well if covered and stored in the refrigerator.

1 cup finely shredded cabbage
½ medium green capsicum, seeded and thinly sliced
½ medium carrot, finely grated
1 medium stick celery, finely chopped
20g sultanas or raisins
1 tablespoon chopped shallots
4 lettuce leaves
For the dressing
1½ tablespoons mayonnaise
2 teaspoons lemon juice
½ teaspoon caraway seeds
salt and pepper

1. Mix the cabbage, green capsicum, carrot, celery, sultanas or raisins and shallots together.

2. Arrange the lettuce leaves around the edge of the serving dish.

3. Stir the dressing ingredients together, pour over the cabbage mixture and toss well to coat all the vegetables.

4. Pile the coleslaw in the centre of the lettuce leaves.

EXCHANGES PER SERVING:
Vegetable 2¾
Fat 3
Fruit ½
25 Kilojoules Optional Exchange

MEDITERRANEAN SALAD

This colorful summer salad, pictured on page 75, makes an enjoyable lunchtime meal.

2 cups cooked elbow macaroni
2 medium tomatoes, coarsely chopped
120g feta cheese, cut into small cubes
¼ cup sliced shallots
3 teaspoons each chopped fresh parsley and basil
2½ tablespoons lemon juice
1 tablespoon olive oil
pinch each salt and pepper
4 pitted black olives, sliced
basil leaves to garnish

1. Mix the macaroni, tomatoes, cheese, shallots, parsley and basil in a bowl.

2. Combine the lemon juice, oil, salt and pepper, pour over salad and toss well.

3. Sprinkle sliced olives over salad just before serving and garnish with basil leaves.

EXCHANGES PER SERVING:
Protein 1
Bread 1
Vegetable 1⅛
Fat 1
10 Kilojoules Optional Exchange

MIXED SALAD WITH BLUE CHEESE DRESSING

SERVES 2

The blue cheese dressing makes almost any salad more tasty and enjoyable. Serve the salad and the dressing separately.

6 medium radicchio leaves
½ medium red or yellow capsicum, seeded and cut in half rings
1 medium stick celery, chopped
1 tablespoon chopped shallots
4 endive leaves
1 small seedless orange
For the dressing
60g blue cheese such as Gorgonzola or Danish Blue
1½-2½ tablespoons cider or white wine vinegar
1 teaspoon olive oil
salt and pepper

1. Place the radicchio leaves, capsicum, celery and shallots in a salad bowl.

2. Tear the endive leaves into pieces and add to the salad.

3. Using a sharp knife, cut the peel and pith off the orange, cut in half lengthwise, then slice. Mix into the salad.

4. Make the dressing. Grate the cheese into a small bowl, mash with a fork and gradually add the vinegar and oil. Season to taste.

5. Serve the salad and dressing separately. Spoon the dressing over the salad just before eating.

EXCHANGES PER SERVING:
Protein 1
Vegetable 1¾
Fat ½
Fruit ½

Mixed Salad with Blue Cheese Dressing.

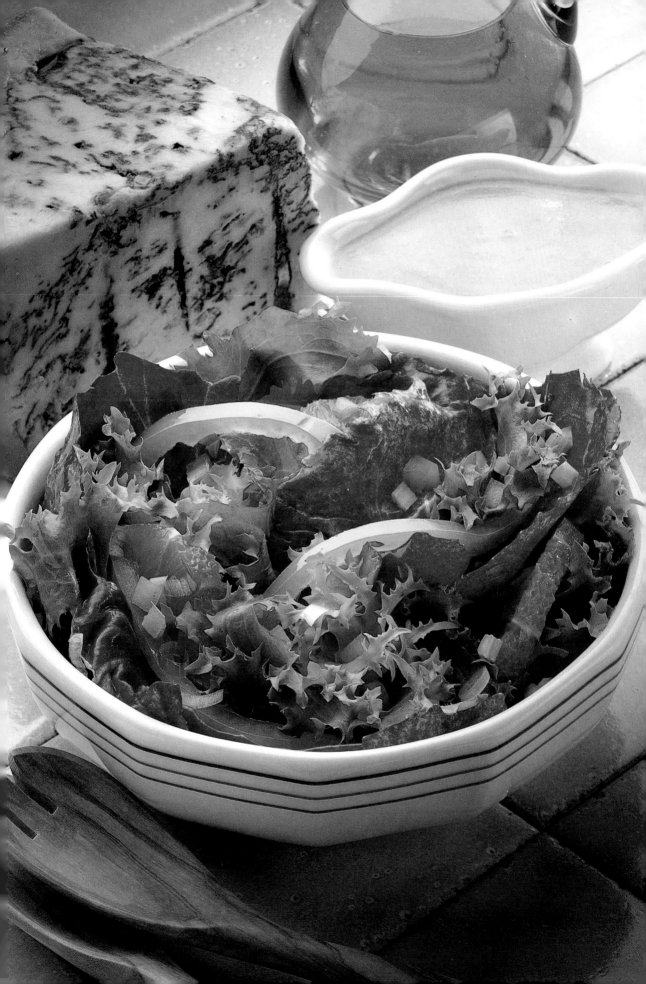

AVOCADO SALAD

SERVES 2

This attractive salad, pictured on page 59, tastes as good as it looks.

1 tablespoon lemon juice
3 teaspoons vegetable oil
1 teaspoon chopped fresh mint
¼ teaspoon each honey and grated orange peel
4 lettuce leaves
50g avocado, thinly sliced
1 small orange, peeled and segmented
¼ cup drained, canned pineapple pieces
6 pecan nuts, roughly chopped
mint leaves to garnish

1. Mix the lemon juice, oil, mint, honey and grated orange peel in a small bowl, cover and refrigerate for 30 minutes.

2. Place lettuce leaves in a serving bowl, arrange avocado slices, orange segments and pineapple pieces in lettuce leaves.

3. Sprinkle with chopped nuts and pour dressing over salad just before serving. Garnish with mint leaves.

EXCHANGES PER SERVING:
Vegetable ½
Fat 1½
Fruit ½
360 Kilojoules Optional Exchange

FRUIT

As the Weight Watchers Food Plan includes a considerable variety of fruit, it's important to include many different kinds in sweet and savory recipes so your diet remains varied and interesting. Always choose good quality fresh fruit.

BRANDIED APRICOTS FLAMBÉ

SERVES 2

This is a dessert for a special occasion — why not flambé the apricots at the table? The cooked apricots in the arrowroot sauce can be used on their own as a stuffing for crepes, page 24, or the brandy may be added to the sauce.

8 medium apricots, halved and stoned
⅓ cup water
1 tablespoon castor sugar
1 teaspoon arrowroot
1½ tablespoons brandy

1. Place the halved apricots and water in a saucepan and heat gently. When the apricots begin to soften, sprinkle in the sugar, cover and simmer over a very low heat until cooked but still whole.

2. Drain the apricots, reserve the syrup, and place in a heatproof dish.

3. Blend the arrowroot with a little of the syrup to form a paste, mix with the remaining syrup and return to the heat. Bring to the boil, stirring all the time, pour the thickened syrup over the apricots.

4. Heat the apricots and syrup over a low heat. Warm the brandy.

5. Remove the apricots from the heat, pour over the brandy and ignite.

EXCHANGES PER SERVING:

Fruit 1
455 Kilojoules Optional Exchange

Brandied Apricots Flambé.

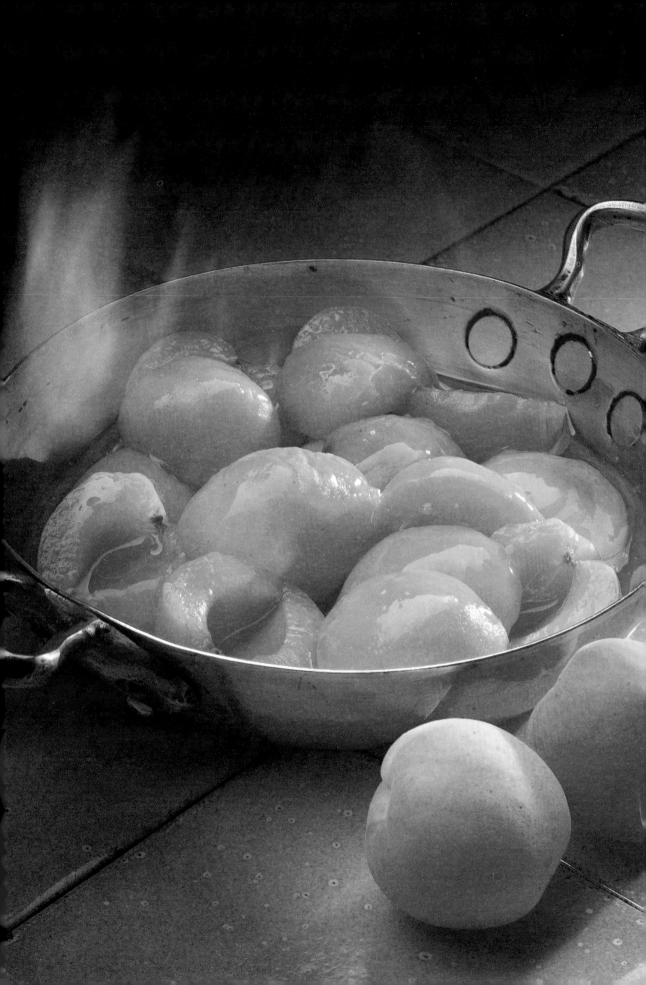

MARINATED FRUITS

This colorful fruit salad makes an attractive dessert suitable for any occasion. Serve on its own, with low-fat natural yoghurt or cream.

200g wedge of honeydew melon or rockmelon
1 large kiwi fruit, sliced
1 medium persimmon, cut in wedges
50g black grapes, halved and seeded
1 large passionfruit
3 teaspoons brandy

1. Cut the melon into chunks or shape into balls using a melon baller or teaspoon.

2. Mix together the melon, kiwi fruit, persimmon and grapes. Scoop out the pulp and seeds from the passionfruit and stir into the other fruits.

3. Sprinkle with brandy. Cover and refrigerate 2-3 hours to marinate before serving.

EXCHANGES PER SERVING:
Fruit 2
80 Kilojoules Optional Exchange

BLACKBERRY APPLE PIE

SERVES 2

The strong flavor of the blackberries combines well with the apples to make a really tasty dessert.

For the pastry
$\frac{1}{3}$ cup plain flour
pinch salt
1 tablespoon polyunsaturated margarine
1-2 teaspoons cold water
For the filling
2 small cooking apples, peeled, quartered, cored and sliced
1 cup frozen blackberries, thawed
2 tablespoons sugar

1. Make the pastry as described on page 108. Cover and leave to rest in the cool while preparing the filling.

2. Arrange half the apples and blackberries in a small pie dish, sprinkle with the sugar and cover with the remaining fruit.

3. Roll out the pastry a little larger than the pie dish, cut off a small strip to just cover the lip of the pie dish. Dampen the pie lip and press the strip of pastry onto the dish. Dampen the pastry edge with cold water and cover with the pastry top, press to seal.

4. Decorate the pastry edge with the prongs of a fork or by pressing the edge with a finger and using the back of the knife to cut through the join several times to form a seal. (A sweet pie does not generally have a fluted edge or a glazed top.) Make a hole in the centre to release the steam while cooking.

5. Place on a baking sheet and bake at 200°C for 15 minutes, then reduce to 170°C for a further 20 minutes to cook the fruit.

EXCHANGES PER SERVING:
Bread 1
Fat 2
Fruit 1½
415 Kilojoules Optional Exchange

BAKED APPLES

—— SERVES 2 ——

This dessert is a longtime favorite and very easy to prepare.

2 small cooking apples
20g raisins
2 teaspoons brown sugar
good pinch mixed spice
2 tablespoons water

1. Wash the apples and remove the cores. Cut 1.25cm off the bottom of each core and replace in the apple to prevent the filling falling out.

2. Cut the skin round the centre of each apple and place in an ovenproof dish.

3. Mix the raisins, sugar and spice together and press into the centre of each apple.

4. Pour the water into the dish and bake at 180°C until the apples are cooked right through, 50-60 minutes.

EXCHANGES PER SERVING:
Fruit 1½
100 Kilojoules Optional Exchange

Baked Apples.

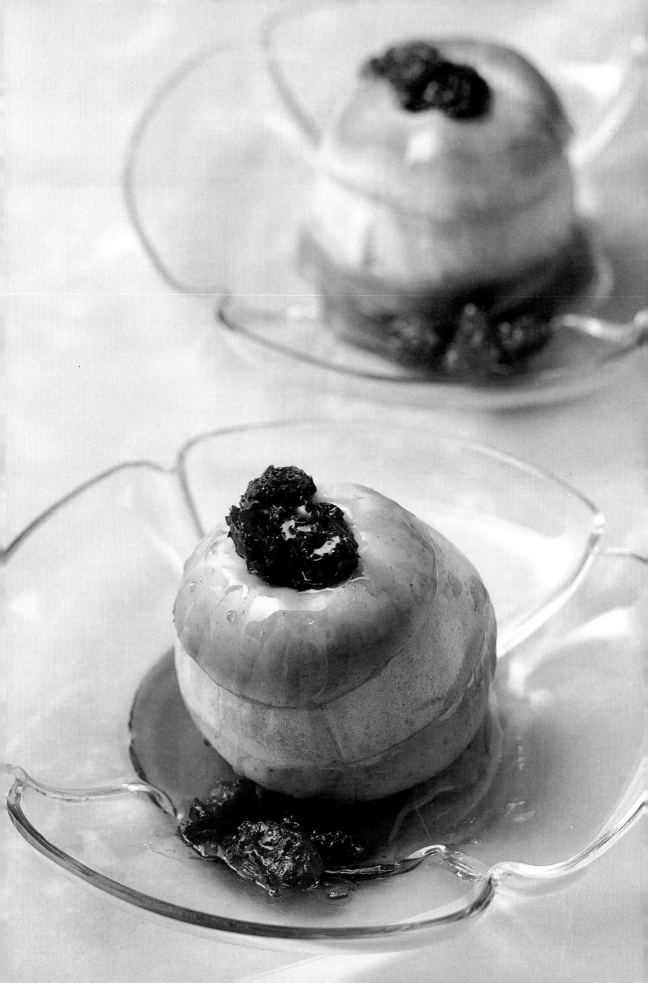

CHERRIES IN RED WINE

Cherries are in season for such a short time so make the most of them. They are delicious in fresh fruit salads, but stewed in red wine they become even more of a treat.

200g red cherries
⅓ cup red wine
1 tablespoon castor sugar
2.5cm cinnamon stick

1. Remove the stalks and stones from the cherries. If you don't possess a cherry stoner, cut each cherry in half and remove the stone. Catch any juices which may drip from the fruit and add to the wine.

2. As the cherries are prepared, drop into the red wine in a saucepan and sprinkle with the castor sugar.

3. Add the cinnamon and bring to the boil, cover, reduce the heat and simmer gently for 10-15 minutes.

4. Serve warm or cool. Remove the cinnamon before serving.

EXCHANGES PER SERVING:
Fruit 1
405 Kilojoules Optional Exchange

PEACH SUNDAE

SERVES 2

It's best to make this dessert, pictured on page 103, when peaches are in season and sweet and juicy. Shredded coconut helps to make this into a pretty dish but it can be difficult to buy. Desiccated coconut tastes equally as good.

2 medium peaches
1 cup frozen raspberries, thawed
1 teaspoon arrowroot
2½ teaspoons sugar
2 teaspoons shredded or desiccated coconut, toasted

1. Pour boiling water over the peaches, leave for 1 minute, plunge into cold water then slip off the skins. Halve and remove the stones.

2. Sieve the raspberries into a saucepan. Blend a little of the raspberry purée into the arrowroot in a bowl. Stir the arrowroot mixture into the rest of the purée, add the sugar and bring to the boil, stirring all the time. Boil for 1 minute, allow to cool.

3. Pour the raspberry sauce over the peaches, divided between two dessert dishes, and sprinkle over the toasted coconut.

EXCHANGES PER SERVING:
Fruit 1½
200 Kilojoules Optional Exchange

SPICED FRUIT COMPÔTE

SERVES 2

As dried fruit is so sweet there is no need for sugar in the syrup.

6 dried apricot halves
3 medium prunes
20g dried apple
½ cup orange juice (no sugar added)
5cm stick of cinnamon
2 whole cloves
2 green cardamoms, seeds removed and pods discarded
zest and juice of ½ a lemon
water, as needed

1. Wash the dried fruit, place in a bowl and add the orange juice and spices.

2. Remove the lemon zest with either a zester or grater, add to the fruits with the lemon juice. Cover, refrigerate and leave to soak overnight.

3. The next day, if necessary, add 1-2 tablespoons water as older dried fruits ab-

sorb more liquid. In a saucepan bring the fruits and spices to the boil, cover and reduce the heat as low as possible. Simmer gently 10-15 minutes until the fruit is cooked.

4. Transfer to a serving bowl and leave to cool or serve warm. Remove the cinnamon stick and other spices before eating.

EXCHANGES PER SERVING:

Fruit 2

Top: Peach Sundae (page 101);
Bottom: Spiced Fruit Compôte.

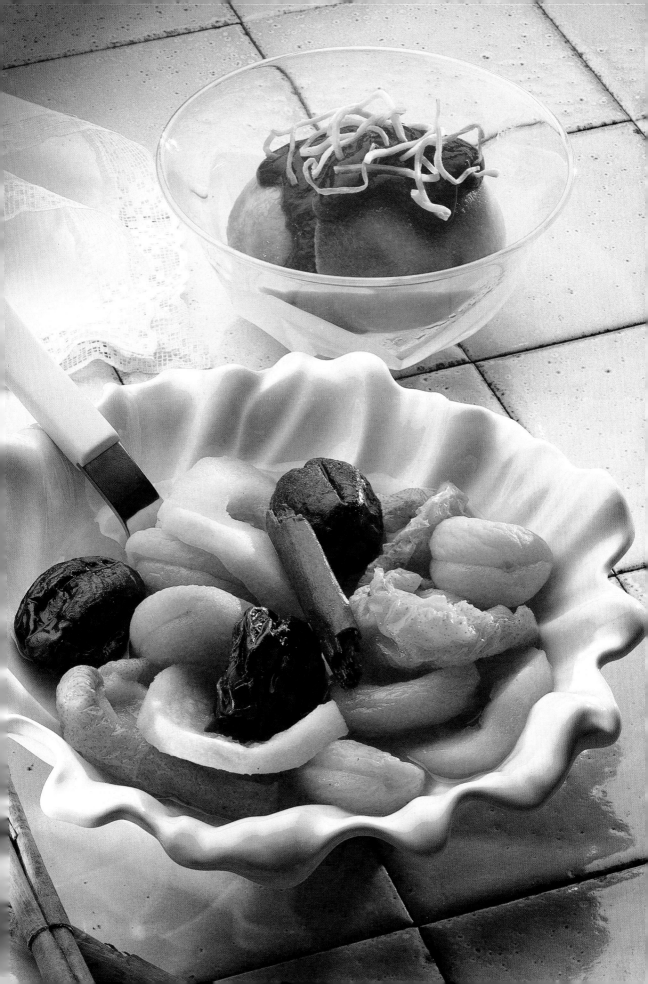

TROPICAL SNOW

— SERVES 2 —

Make this dessert and serve immediately. If it's made too far in advance, the egg white foam will gradually collapse.

½ small mango, peeled and seeded
½ small banana, peeled
2-3 teaspoons lemon juice
1½ teaspoons castor sugar
finely grated zest of ½ a lemon
1 egg white
2 lemon slices for garnish.

1. Mash the mango, banana, lemon juice, sugar and lemon zest.

2. Whisk the egg white in a bowl until soft peaks form.

3. Add the fruit purée to the egg white and whisk again to form a foam. Pile the snow into two serving dishes and serve garnished with lemon slices.

EXCHANGES PER SERVING:

Fruit ½

180 Kilojoules Optional Exchange

BAKING

This chapter includes pastries, biscuits, cakes, scones and bread. The main in-gredients used for baking are flour, fat, sugar, eggs, liquid and flavorings. Each ingredient has a particular function to perform and the quantity and method by which it is incorporated into the recipe affects the end result.

FRUIT TARTS

Almost any fruit can be served in this way and, as a treat, can be enjoyed with cream or thawed frozen whipped topping.

For the pastry
⅓ cup plain flour
pinch salt
1 tablespoon polyunsaturated margarine
1-2 teaspoons cold water
For the filling
2 medium dessert plums, stoned and cut into wedges or 3 medium apricots, stoned and cut into wedges or 1 cup strawberries, halved
For the glaze
¼ cup fresh orange juice
1 teaspoon arrowroot
1 teaspoon sugar

1. Make the pastry as described on page 108.

2. Roll out and line two 9cm fluted flan cases. Prick the pastry bases. Cut two circles of baking paper a little larger than the flan cases. Place each circle of paper in the pastry case and weigh down with a few dried beans. Transfer to a hot baking sheet and bake at 200°C for 10 minutes, remove the paper and beans and return to the oven for a further 4-5 minutes. Leave to cool.

3. Arrange the fruit decoratively in the pastry cases.

4. Make the glaze. In a small bowl blend half of the orange juice with the arrowroot to a paste. Pour the orange juice mixture, remaining orange juice and sugar into a very small saucepan. Bring to the boil, stirring all the time. Boil for 1 minute.

5. Brush the glaze over the fruit.

EXCHANGES PER SERVING:
Bread 1
Fat 2
Fruit ½
140 Kilojoules Optional Exchange

Fruit Tarts.

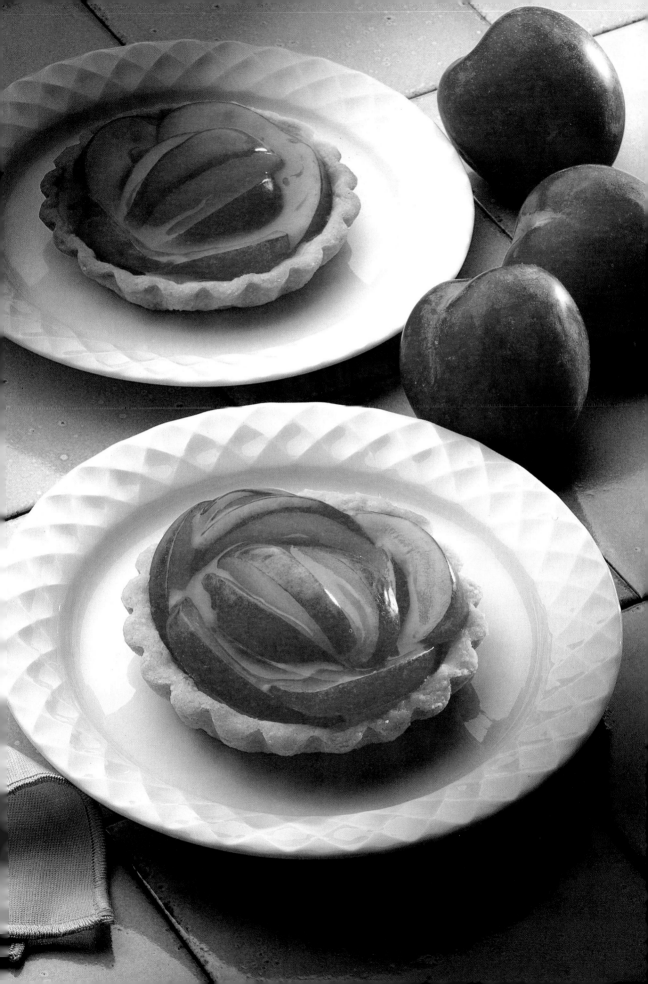

SHORTCRUST PASTRY

SERVES 2

This pastry is used in recipes in this book but the guidelines given here should always be followed.

⅓ cup plain flour
pinch salt
1 tablespoon polyunsaturated margarine
1-2 teaspoons ice-cold water

1. Sieve the flour and salt into a small bowl. Reserve 2 teaspoons of flour mixture.

2. Add the margarine, if possible margarine which has been stored in the freezer. Rub into the flour mixture using the tips of your fingers and thumbs.

3. Mix the cold water into the pastry with a round bladed knife. If time allows, wrap in foil or plastic foodwrap and refrigerate for 15-20 minutes.

4. Dust the work surface and rolling pin with the reserved flour. Roll out the pastry using short, light movements away from you. Turn the pastry to roll to the correct shape. Don't alter the movement of the rolling as this will stretch the pastry and cause it to shrink during cooking.

5. Bake according to the recipe, usually between 190-200°C for the first 15 minutes. If using the pastry for flans or pastry bases, it is worth standing the pie or flan plate on a baking sheet which has been heated in the oven. This helps the pastry to bake evenly and not become soggy on the bottom.

EXCHANGES PER SERVING:
Bread 1
Fat 2
15 Kilojoules Optional Exchange

SULTANA CAKES

These small cakes, pictured on page 123, are very easy to make. Try adding a little mixed spice or ground ginger to the flour.

60g polyunsaturated margarine
¼ cup castor sugar
1 egg, beaten
40g sultanas
¾ cup self-raising flour

1. Arrange 10 paper cake cases in a patty cake pan.

2. Cream the margarine and sugar until light and fluffy, add the egg a teaspoon at a time and beat well after each addition.

3. Fold the sultanas into the creamed mix-ture, then sieve the flour and fold into the mixture using a metal spoon.

4. Divide the mixture between the cake cases and bake at 190°C for 15-20 minutes. Cool on a wire rack.

FRUIT RINGS

SERVES 2

It's hard to believe that you can be following a slimming diet and still enjoy a dessert like this one. It's important to make a slit in the choux pastry to allow the steam to escape or the pastry will be soggy.

For the choux pastry
3 tablespoons water
1 tablespoon polyunsaturated margarine
¼ cup plain flour, sieved
1 egg, beaten
For the filling
1 large kiwi fruit, sliced and halved
1 cup strawberries or raspberries, halved
30g thawed frozen whipped topping
½ teaspoon icing sugar to dust the tops

1. Line a baking sheet with baking paper.

2. Make the pastry. Gently heat the water and margarine in a saucepan until the margarine has melted. Increase the heat and bring to a rolling boil. Tip in all the flour and beat well over a moderate heat for 1 minute. By this time the mixture will be in a ball. Allow to cool a little and then gradually add the egg, beating well after each addition.

3. Preheat oven to 200°C. Using a 1.25cm plain nozzle, pipe a 7.5cm circle on the prepared baking sheet. Pipe another circle on top of the first. Repeat this procedure to form two rings.

4. Place the choux rings in the oven and immediately increase the heat to 220°C. Cook for 30 minutes until well risen and golden brown. Make a slit in each ring to allow the steam to escape. Return to the oven for a further 5 minutes. Cool on a wire rack.

5. No more than half an hour before serving, cut horizontally through each choux ring. Arrange half of the kiwi fruit slices on each bottom ring, top each with half of the strawberries or raspberries, then half of the thawed frozen whipped topping. Cover with the top of the choux ring and dust with icing sugar. If there are any strawberries or raspberries left over, pile them in the centre.

EXCHANGES PER SERVING:
Protein ½
Bread ½
Fat 2
Fruit 1
340 Kilojoules Optional Exchange

Fruit Rings.

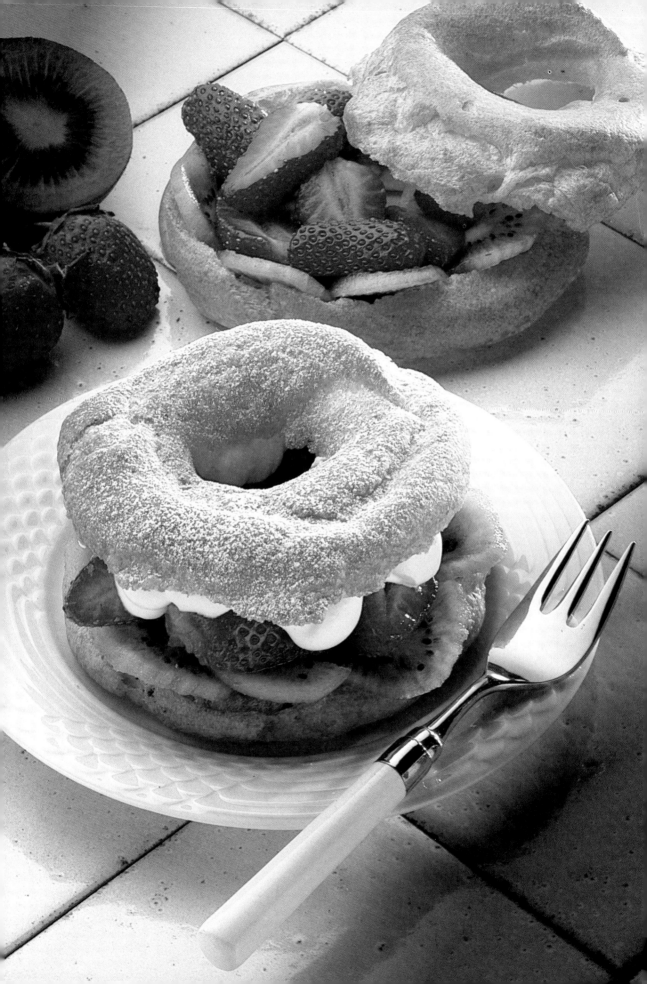

BASIC BREAD LOAF

MAKES 1 LARGE OR 2 SMALL LOAVES

This recipe, pictured on page 123, can be used to make white, grain or wholemeal bread and it can easily be adapted to shape into a plait or cottage loaf. To make a savory loaf to serve with soups, add 3-4 tablespoons of freshly chopped mixed herbs to the flour.

1 teaspoon sugar
1¾ cups warm water
3 teaspoons dried yeast
6 cups wholemeal, grain or plain flour
2 teaspoons salt
3 teaspoons polyunsaturated margarine
1 teaspoon oil

1. Dissolve the sugar into the water, add the yeast and stir until dissolved. Leave in a warm place for 10-15 minutes or until frothy.

2. Reserve a tablespoon of flour. Stir the remaining flour and salt together in a bowl, rub in the margarine.

3. Add the yeast liquid to the flour and mix to form a firm dough, add a little extra warm water if necessary.

4. Use the reserved flour to lightly dust the work surface. Knead the dough on the floured surface for about 10 minutes until smooth and elastic. (If you have a food processor or mixer with a dough attachment, this can be achieved in 2-3 minutes.)

5. Place the dough in a clean bowl, lightly grease a sheet of plastic foodwrap with ¼ teaspoon oil and use to cover the dough. Leave in a warm place until the dough has doubled in size. Meanwhile, use the remaining oil to grease a 1kg loaf pan or two 500g loaf pans.

6. Turn the dough out and knead for 2-3 minutes. Shape to fit the prepared pan or pans, cover with the oiled plastic foodwrap and leave in the warm to prove. The dough should rise to the top of the pan and when lightly pressed with a finger should spring back.

7. Bake in a preheated oven, 230°C allowing about 30 minutes for the smaller loaves and about 35 minutes for the large loaf.

8. Turn the bread out of the pan and tap the base — it should sound hollow when cooked. Leave to cool on a wire rack.

EXCHANGES PER SERVING:
Use as for ordinary Bread Exchanges
(i.e. 30g slice = 1 Bread Exchange).

NUTTY DAMPER

A damper with a difference. A nice accompaniment to the Veal Roast, both pictured on page 55.

1 teaspoon polyunsaturated margarine
3 cups self-raising flour
⅓ cup peanut butter
1¼ cups skim milk
2 teaspoons plain flour

1. Grease the base of a 20cm spring-form cake pan with the margarine.

2. Sift flour into a bowl. Rub in the peanut butter until the mixture resembles fresh breadcrumbs.

3. Make a well in the centre of the flour, add the milk and mix to form a slightly sticky dough with a round-bladed knife.

4. Preheat oven to 190°C. Knead lightly to form dough into a ball. Place dough on prepared pan and sprinkle with plain flour.

5. Bake for about 30 minutes or until damper sounds hollow when tapped.

EXCHANGES PER SERVING:
Protein ½
Bread 2
Fat ½
320 Kilojoules Optional Exchange

FILLED CHEESE SCONES

SERVES 8

This recipe uses Cheddar cheese in the scone dough and the filling but it is worth changing the filling cheese to add variety.

For the scones
2 cups plain flour
2½ teaspoons baking powder
½ teaspoon powdered mustard
¼ teaspoon salt
2 tablespoons polyunsaturated margarine
90g Cheddar cheese, finely grated
⅔ cup skim milk

For the filling
240g ricotta cheese
90g Cheddar cheese, grated
½ teaspoon chilli sauce
4 lettuce leaves
2 medium tomatoes, sliced
½ cup sliced cucumber
celery leaf to garnish

1. Line a baking sheet with baking paper.

2. Reserve 2 teaspoons flour. Sieve the remaining flour, baking powder, mustard and salt into a bowl. Rub in the margarine until the mixture resembles fresh breadcrumbs. Stir in the finely grated cheese.

3. Make a well in the centre of the flour, add most of the milk and mix to form a soft dough with a round bladed knife. Add remaining milk, reserving 1 teaspoon of milk for glazing.

4. Sprinkle the work surface with the reserved flour and lightly dust the rolling pin. Roll out the dough to form a circle, 2cm thick.

5. Transfer the scone to the lined baking sheet, brush with the teaspoon of milk and mark into eight wedges but leave in one piece. Leave to stand 15-20 minutes.

6. Bake in a preheated oven at 230°C for 15-20 minutes until well risen, golden and cooked through. Cool on a wire rack.

7. While the scones are cooling, mix together the cheeses and season with chilli sauce.

8. Cut the scones in half horizontally. Spread half of the cheese filling over cut side of each half. Arrange the lettuce, tomato and cucumber on the bottom half, replace the top and cut into eight portions.

EXCHANGES PER SERVING:
Protein 1
Bread 1½
Vegetable ¾
Fat 1
135 Kilojoules Optional Exchange

Filled Cheese Scones, seven serving pictured

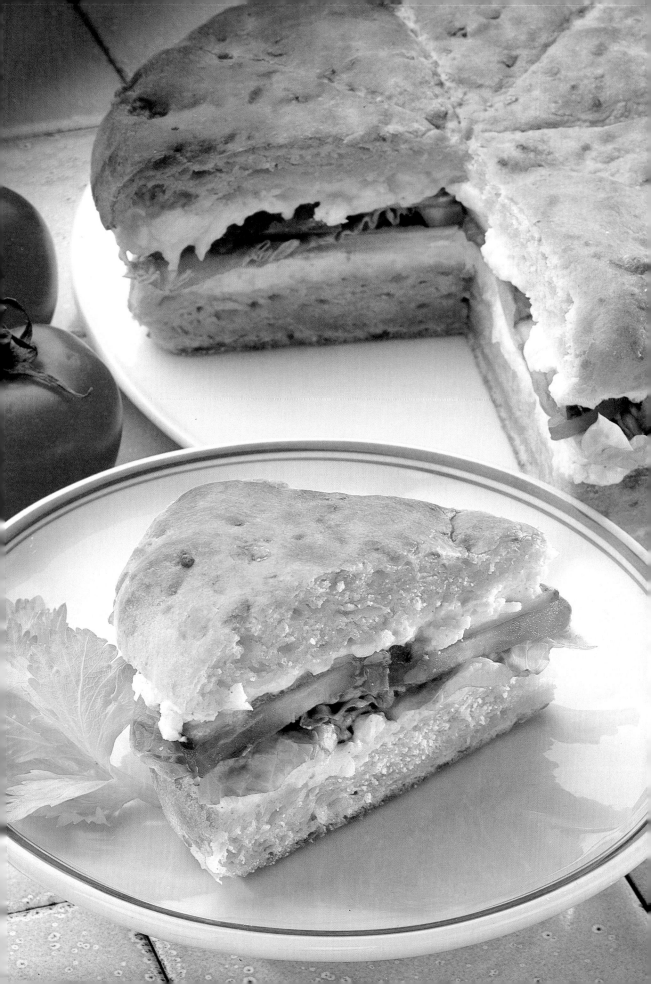

SHORTBREAD BISCUITS

SERVES 12

Keep a vanilla pod in a jar of castor sugar for using when cake and biscuit making. It eliminates the need for vanilla essence and imparts a delicate flavor to sauces and desserts as well. This recipe is pictured on page 119.

60g polyunsaturated margarine
1½ tablespoons castor sugar
few drops of vanilla essence
¾ cup plain flour

1. Line a baking sheet with baking paper.

2. Cream the margarine and castor sugar together, add the vanilla essence.

3. Reserve 2 teaspoons flour. Stir the remaining flour into the creamed margarine to form a soft dough.

4. Sprinkle the reserved flour over the work surface and rolling pin. Roll out the dough to about 5mm thick, cut into 12 biscuits using a 6.5cm cutter. Re-roll the trimmings as necessary.

5. Place the biscuits on the prepared baking sheet and prick with a fork. Bake at 160°C for about 15 minutes until lightly browned. Cool on a wire rack.

EXCHANGES PER SERVING:

Fat 1
205 Kilojoules Optional Exchange

GINGERNUTS

SERVES 12

These crunchy little biscuits, pictured on page 119, are made using the melting method. When rolling into small balls and flattening before baking, don't try to smooth out the cracks, these are characteristic of the biscuits.

1 cup self-raising flour
2 teaspoons ground ginger
½ teaspoon bicarbonate of soda
¼ teaspoon ground cinnamon
60g polyunsaturated margarine
1½ tablespoons brown sugar
3 teaspoons clear honey

1. Line a baking sheet with baking paper.

2. Sieve the flour, ginger, bicarbonate of soda and cinnamon into a bowl.

3. In a saucepan gently heat the margarine, sugar and honey until the margarine has melted and the sugar dissolved.

4. Pour the margarine mixture into the flour and mix well.

5. Divide into 12 pieces and roll into small balls, place on the lined baking sheet and flatten with the palm of your hand.

6. Bake 180°C for about 15 minutes. Cool on a wire rack.

EXCHANGES PER SERVING:
Bread ½
Fat 1
85 Kilojoules Optional Exchange

SPEEDY SANDWICH CAKE

SERVES 12

This simple recipe is ideal if you are expecting visitors at short notice. In a matter of minutes the ingredients can be weighed out, beaten and the cake is ready for baking.

½ teaspoon vegetable oil
½ cup castor sugar
120g polyunsaturated margarine
2 eggs
½ teaspoon grated lemon zest
1 cup self-raising flour
1 teaspoon baking powder
2 tablespoons raspberry or strawberry jam
½ teaspoon icing sugar, sieved

1. Oil each of two 16cm sandwich pans with half of the oil and line the bases with baking paper.

2. Preheat oven to 170-180°C. Place the castor sugar, margarine, eggs and lemon zest into a bowl. Sieve in the flour and baking powder and beat all the ingredients together, using a wooden spoon, for about 1½ minutes.

3. Divide the mixture between the prepared pans, level the surfaces and bake for 25-30 minutes. Allow to cool for 2-3 minutes, then turn out onto a cooling rack and leave until cold.

4. Sandwich the cakes together with the jam and dust the top with the sieved icing sugar.

EXCHANGES PER SERVING:
Bread ½
Fat 2
320 Kilojoules Optional Exchange

Top: Gingernuts (page 117);
Speedy Sandwich Cake;
Centre: Shortbread Biscuits (page 116);
Bottom: Flapjacks (page 121).

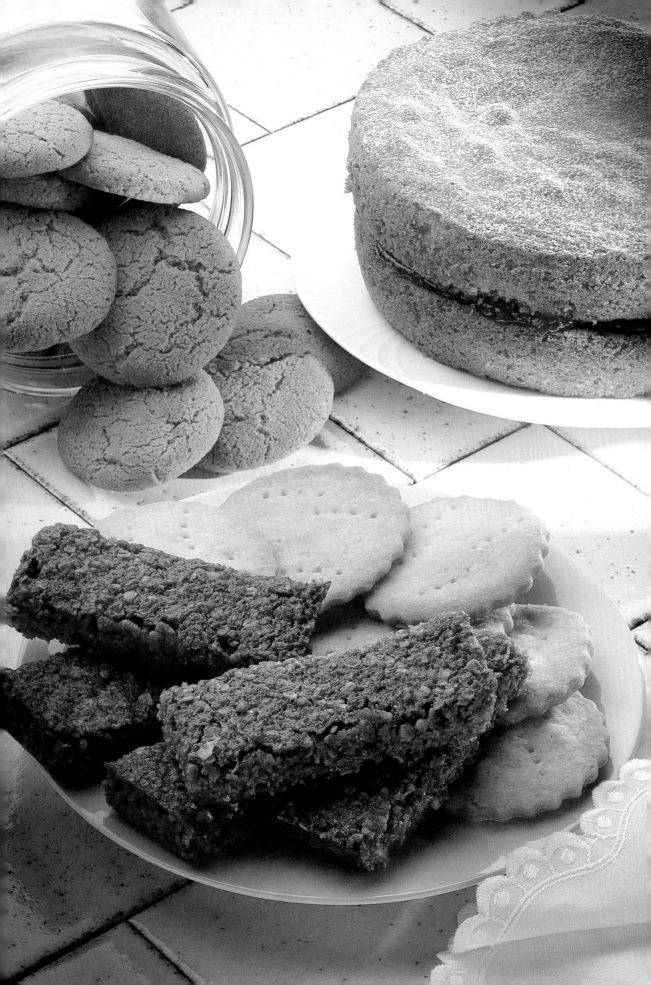

FRUIT BUNS

SERVES 12

These fruit buns, pictured on page 123, can easily be made into spicy hot cross buns. Add an extra ½ teaspoon mixed spice then, just before baking, mark the top of each bun with a cross.

⅔ cup skim milk

¼ cup water

1½ tablespoons castor sugar

3 teaspoons dried yeast

4 cups plain flour

1½ teaspoons salt

1 teaspoon mixed spice

60g polyunsaturated margarine

120g mixed dried fruit

1 egg, beaten

For the glaze

2 tablespoons water

1 tablespoon sugar

1. Line two baking sheets with non-stick paper.

2. Gently heat the milk and water until warm, dissolve 1 teaspoon castor sugar in the liquid, sprinkle in the yeast and mix well. Leave in a warm place for 10-15 minutes until frothy.

3. Reserve a tablespoon of flour. Sieve the flour, salt and spice into a bowl.

4. Spray a sheet of plastic foodwrap with non-stick cooking spray. Rub the margarine into the flour. Stir in the dried fruit.

5. Pour the yeast liquid into the flour and mix to form a firm dough, adding all but 1 tablespoon of the beaten egg. Do not discard the remaining egg.

6. Use the reserved flour to lightly dust the work surface. Knead the dough on the floured surface for about 10 minutes until smooth and elastic. (If you have a food processor or mixer with a dough attachment, this can be achieved in 2-3 minutes.)

7. Place the dough in a clean bowl and re-cover with sprayed plastic foodwrap. Leave in a warm place until the dough has doubled in size.

8. Turn the dough out and knead for 2-3 minutes. Divide into 12 pieces, roll each into a ball and place well spaced out on the prepared baking sheets. Cover with the sprayed plastic foodwrap and leave in the warm to prove. The buns should almost double in size. Brush buns with remaining beaten egg, be sure to use all of the egg.

9. Bake in a preheated oven 230°C for about 15 minutes. Cool on a wire rack.

10. While the buns are cooking, make the sugar glaze. Place the water and sugar in a small saucepan, heat gently until the sugar has dissolved, then increase the heat and boil fiercely for 1 minute. Brush the warm buns with the hot glaze.

EXCHANGES PER SERVING:
Bread 2
Fat 1
Fruit ½
165 Kilojoules Optional Exchange

FLAPJACKS

These biscuits, pictured on page 119, are rather more-ish so it is best to store them in a tin out of temptation's way.

$\frac{1}{2}$ cup brown sugar
120g polyunsaturated margarine
3 teaspoons golden syrup
240g rolled oats
$\frac{1}{2}$ teaspoon ground allspice

1. Line a 18x28cm Swiss roll pan with baking paper.

2. Gently heat the sugar, margarine and syrup in a saucepan.

3. Preheat oven to 190°C. When the margarine has melted, stir in the oats and spice, mix well.

4. Transfer the mixture to the prepared pan and press down to level the surface.

5. Bake for 20-25 minutes until golden brown. Mark into 12 fingers and leave in the tin to cool.

EXCHANGES PER SERVING:
Bread 1
Fat 2
235 Kilojoules Optional Exchange

WHOLEGRAIN KNOTS

SERVES 9

Although this recipe describes how to shape lengths of dough in knot-shaped rolls, other shapes can also be made. With other shapes it is best to dampen the end of the dough with a little water and press to the main shape. Be sure to weigh roll before serving.

½ teaspoon vegetable oil
¾ cup warm skim milk
1 teaspoon sugar
2 teaspoons dried yeast
360g wholegrain plain flour
1 teaspoon salt
3 teaspoons polyunsaturated margarine

1. Line a baking sheet with baking paper. Brush a piece of plastic foodwrap with the oil.

2. Place the warm milk in a jug, dissolve the sugar in the milk, then add the yeast and stir until dissolved. Leave in a warm place for 10-15 minutes or until frothy.

3. Reserve a tablespoon of flour. Stir the remaining flour and salt together in a bowl, rub in the margarine.

4. Add the yeast liquid to the flour and mix to form a firm dough.

5. Use the reserved flour to lightly dust the work surface. Knead the dough on the floured surface for about 10 minutes until smooth and elastic. (If you have a food processor or mixer with a dough attachment, this can be achieved in 2-3 minutes.)

6. Place the dough in a clean bowl, cover with the oiled plastic foodwrap and leave in a warm place until the dough has doubled in size.

7. Turn the dough out and knead for 2-3 minutes. Divide into 9 equal pieces and roll each piece into a long length, tie loosely into a knot and place on the lined baking sheet. Cover with the oiled plastic foodwrap and leave to prove until almost double in size.

8. Bake at 230°C for about 15 minutes. Leave to cool on a wire rack.

EXCHANGES PER SERVING:
Use as for ordinary Bread Exchanges (i.e. 30g slice = 1 Bread Exchange).

Top: Fruit Buns (page 120);
Basic Bread Loaf;
Centre: Wholegrain Knots (page 122);
Bottom: Sultana Cakes (page 109).

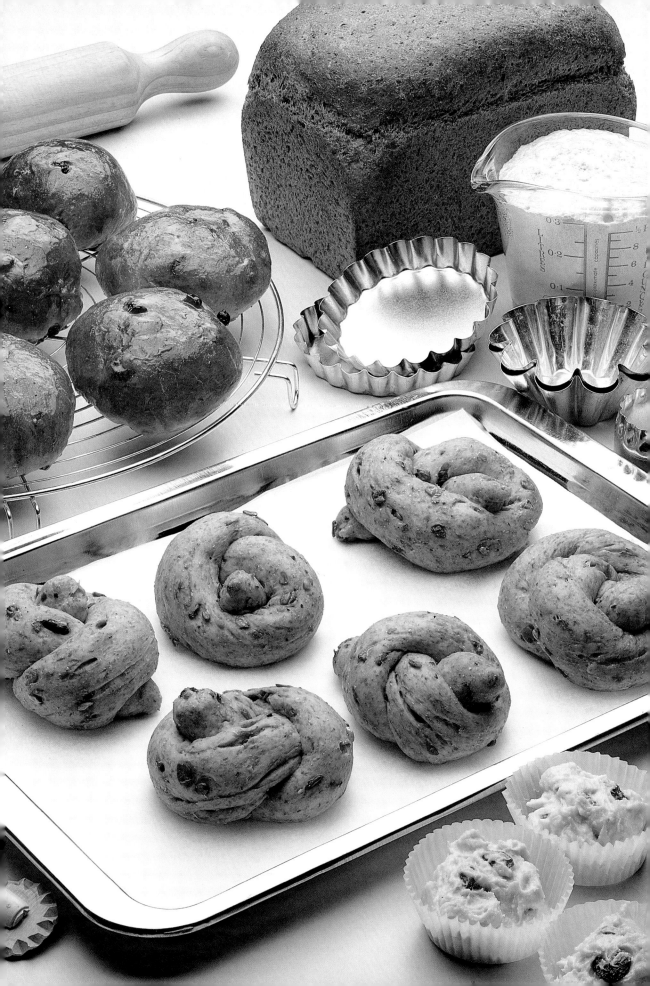

INDEX